THE CULTURAL CONTEXT OF THERAPEUTIC CHOICE

CULTURE, ILLNESS, AND HEALING

Studies in Comparative Cross-Cultural Research

VOLUME 3

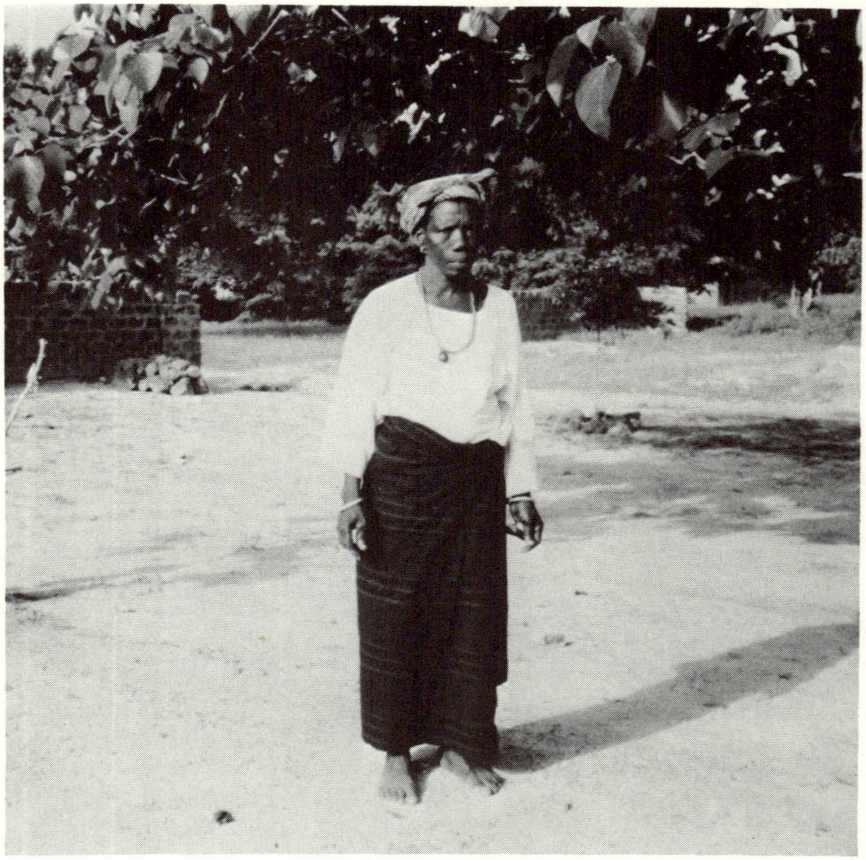

Yaayi Yo, Bariba Midwife.

THE CULTURAL CONTEXT OF THERAPEUTIC CHOICE

Obstetrical Care Decisions Among the Bariba of Benin

by

CAROLYN FISHEL SARGENT

Department of Anthropology, Southern Methodist University, Dallas, U.S.A.

D. REIDEL PUBLISHING COMPANY

DORDRECHT : HOLLAND / BOSTON : U.S.A.

LONDON : ENGLAND

Library of Congress Cataloging in Publication Data

CIP

Sargent, Carolyn Fishel, 1947–
The cultural context of therapeutic choice.

(Culture, illness, and healing ; v. 3)
Bibliography: p.
Includes index.
1. Bariba (African people)–Medicine. 2. Birth customs–Benin. 3. Midwives–Benin. 4. Maternal health services–Benin. I. Title. II. Series. [DNLM: 1. Midwifery–Africa, Western. 2. Medicine, Traditional–Africa, Western. 3. Culture. 4. Maternal health services–Africa, Western. W1 CU445 v. 3 / WQ 160 S245c]
DT541.45.B37S257 362.1'98200966'83 81-23473
ISBN 90-277-1344-8 AACR2

Published by D. Reidel Publishing Company,
P.O. Box 17, 3300 AA Dordrecht, Holland.

Sold and distributed in the U.S.A. and Canada
by Kluwer Boston Inc.,
190 Old Derby Street, Hingham, MA 02043, U.S.A.

In all other countries, sold and distributed
by Kluwer Academic Publishers Group,
P.O. Box 322, 3300 AH Dordrecht, Holland.

D. Reidel Publishing Company is a member of the Kluwer Group.

Printed in The Netherlands

TABLE OF CONTENTS

PREFACE xi

CHAPTER 1: INTRODUCTION 1
1.1. The Study 1
1.2. The Setting 3
1.3. Methodology 5
1.4. Theoretical Perspectives on Health Care Decisions 8

CHAPTER 2: THE CULTURAL CONTEXT OF THERAPEUTIC CHOICE 19
2.1. Bariba Conceptions of the Order of the Universe 19
2.2. Diagnosis and Treatment 24
2.3. Divination 28
2.4. The Use of Substances 30
2.5. Medicines 32

CHAPTER 3: BELIEFS AND PRACTICES SURROUNDING REPRODUCTIVE PROCESSES 35
3.1. Menstruation and Clitoridectomy 35
3.2. Conception 37
3.3. Development of Fetus 39
3.4. Contraception 39
3.5. Abortion 40
3.6. Sterility 41

CHAPTER 4: STATUS AMONG THE BARIBA: THE ROLES AND RESPONSIBILITIES OF WOMEN 43
4.1. Status in Bariba Society 44
4.2. Position of Women 46
4.3. Economic Subsistence 46
4.4. Political Arena 49
4.5. Domestic Relations 50
4.5.1. Marriage 50
4.6. Household Responsibilities 51

CHAPTER 5: SOCIOLOGICAL AND CAREER ATTRIBUTES OF MIDWIVES 56
5.1. Healers: Midwives and Medicine People 56

5.1.1. *Tingi*: The Medicine Person 56
5.1.2. Apprenticeship 58
5.1.3. The Power of Words 59
5.1.4. Midwife as Healer 60
5.1.5. Midwife as a Category 61
5.2. Implications of Role Expectations for Birth Assistance 62
5.2.1. Status Characteristics of Midwives 63
5.2.1.1. Religion 63
5.2.1.2. Age 64
5.2.1.3. Birth and Residence 64
5.2.1.4. Education 64
5.2.1.5. Marital Status 65
5.2.1.6. Occupation of Husband 66
5.2.1.7. Family Origin 66
5.3. Recruitment of Matrones and Method of Skill Acquisition 67
5.4. Sources of Medical Knowledge 69
5.5. Matrones Own Reproductive Histories 70
5.6. Age at Unsupervised Delivery 70
5.7. Assistance at Own Child's Delivery 71
5.8. Remuneration 71
5.9. Comprehensive Care by Matrones 74
5.10. Pregnancy Counseling 75
5.11. Matrone's Role Variability 76
5.12. Spirit Possession 77
5.13. Inheritance of Spirits 79
5.14. Healing and Sambani 80
5.15. The Matrone Prototype 82

CHAPTER 6: THE MEANING OF EFFICACY IN RELATION TO OBSTETRICAL CARE PREFERENCES 86

CHAPTER 7: BIRTH ASSISTANCE IN THE RURAL AREA: PATTERNS OF DELIVERY ASSISTANCE 96
7.1. Delivery Assistance: Patterns of Selection in the Rural Area 96
7.1.1. Person Present at Last Delivery 97
7.1.2. Clients and Cord-Cutters 99
7.1.3. The Baby-Washer 101
7.2. Midwifery as a Therapeutic System 105
7.3. Structured Interviews with Matrones 106

CHAPTER 8: CLIENT-PRACTITIONER ENCOUNTERS 111
8.1.1. The Case of Adama 111
8.1.1.1. Comments 113
8.1.2. The Case of Sako 114

8.1.2.1. Comments 115
8.1.3. The Case of the Prolapsed Cord 116
8.1.3.1. Comments 118
8.1.4. The Case of the Terrifying Breech 120
8.1.4.1. Comments 120
8.1.5. The Case of Bona 120
8.1.5.1. Comments 123
8.2. Pain as a Cultural Phenomenon 124
8.3. Pregnancy (by Nicole) 131
8.4. Conclusion 131

CHAPTER 9: UTILIZATION OF NATIONAL HEALTH SERVICES FOR MATERNITY CARE IN THE DISTRICT OF KOUANDE 134
9.1. Clinic vs. Home Delivery: A Pehunko Sample 134
9.2. Utilization of the Pehunko Dispensary 134
9.2.1. Summary Points 136
9.3. Pehunko Women at the Kouande Maternity Clinic 137
9.3.1. Summary Points 137
9.4. The Kouande Maternity Clinic: General Utilization 138
9.4.1. Distance 138
9.4.2. Prenatal Consultations 140
9.4.3. Reasons for Utilizing the Clinic 141
9.4.4. Features of the Model 144
9.4.5. Morbidity and Mortality 146
9.4.6. The Etic Perspective 147
9.4.7. The Clinic Setting 151
9.4.8. The Emic Perspective 155

CHAPTER 10: CONCLUSION 157
10.1. Implications of the Bariba Study for the Cross-Cultural Study of Midwifery 157
10.2. The Involvement of Indigenous Midwives in National Health Systems 159
10.3. Training Programs 163

APPENDICES 168
Appendix A: Demographic Data 168
Appendix B: Female Circumcision Songs 169

NOTES 171

BIBLIOGRAPHY 178

INDEX 186

PREFACE

This book examines the factors influencing women's choices of obstetrical care in a Bariba community in the People's Republic of Benin, West Africa. When selecting a research topic, I decided to investigate health care among the Bariba for several reasons. First, I had served as a Peace Corps Volunteer in northern Benin (then Dahomey) and had established a network of contacts in the region. In addition, I had worked for a year as assistant manager of a pharmacy in a northern town and had become interested in the pattern of utilization of health care services by urban residents. This three-year residence proved an invaluable asset in preparing and conducting research in the northern region. In particular, I was able to establish relationships with several indigenous midwives whose families I already knew both from prior research experience and mutual friendships. These relationships enabled me to obtain detailed information regarding obstetrical practice and thus form the foundation of this book.

The fieldwork upon which the book is directly based was conducted between June 1976 and December 1977 and sponsored by the Ford-Rockefeller Population Policy Program, the Social Science Research Council, the National Science Foundation, and the Fulbright-Hays Doctoral Dissertation Research Program. The Ford-Rockefeller Population Policy Program funded the project as a collaboration between myself and Professor Eusèbe Alihonou, Professor Agrégé (Gynécologie-Obstétrique) at the National University of Benin.

I am especially indebted to Dr. Alihonou for his assistance in designing the research and in editing and analyzing medical data, and for his efforts to arrange prenatal consultations at the fieldwork site of Pehunko. In addition, I am grateful to the Ministry of Health of the People's Republic of Benin and to the National University of Benin for enabling me to pursue this project. Dr. Cecile De Sweemer, then Program Advisor for Health and Family Planning for the Ford Foundation West Africa Regional Office provided support and organizational assistance throughout the fieldwork period, for which I remain appreciative, and Father Daniel Cardot generously allowed me to study his notebooks on Bariba tradition which he has collected over more than ten years in Benin.

I am also grateful to Arthur J. Rubel, John Hinnant, John M. Hunter, and Brigitte Jordan, who provided me with direction and advice during the preparation of this study, to Harry Raulet and Robert McKinley for their longstanding interest in my work, to Robert Van Kemper, for editorial assistance, and to Linda Whiteford for her unflagging reassurance. In addition, I would like to acknowledge the help of Arthur Kleinman, whose careful scrutiny of several versions of this manuscript aided in consolidating my thinking on numerous points, and I thank Sheryl St. Germain and Kathleen Triplett who efficiently typed several manuscript drafts.

Finally, I wish to express particular gratitude to my family for their encouragement throughout my graduate studies, and to Kora Zaki Zaliatou, my neighbor in the village of Pehunko, whose pithy comments regarding anthropological research, Bariba culture, and the meaning of being a woman made my research both a professionally rewarding and personally enriching experience.

CHAPTER 1

INTRODUCTION

Throughout the Third World, a notable trend has been the proliferation of parallel health care systems in which cosmopolitan medical services coexist with a variety of indigenous health care services. Among the most ubiquitous of such services are those which provide maternal and child health care. Within the domain of maternal and child health services, an increasing number of options are available to client populations, including hospitals, private clinics, missionary health services, indigenous herbalists, diviners, midwives, injection dealers; hence decisions must be made regarding the preferred choice among the existing alternatives. Alternative utilization of maternal and child health services, and in particular, obstetrical services, represents one arena within which to study health care decision-making. Obstetrical care is broadly defined here to encompass prenatal care, delivery assistance and postpartum care, fertility counseling and infant care, and thus refers to a range of widely sought after services.

A consideration of the utilization of obstetrical services in an area such as rural Africa highlights a number of significant issues. Among these are the delineation of patterns of utilization of cosmopolitan and indigenous practitioners; the efficacy of different alternatives (including modes of measuring or evaluating 'efficacy'); and the role for indigenous healers in national health plans. All of the above issues are relevant to determining the most feasible methods of delivering optimum health care to rural African populations.

An additional topic of significance which is related to the utilization of obstetrical services in rural Africa is the role of women in the household, as professional specialists, and in society in general. In the West African setting, childbearing is fundamental to a woman's status, and reproduction is thus of particular concern to women. Moreover, specialists dealing with reproductive functions tend to be female. Research on factors influencing choices of obstetrical assistance, then, has implications for the study of decision-making, the provision of health care to rural African populations, the cross-cultural study of the status of women, and the study of indigenous midwifery.

1.1. THE STUDY

This book explains the factors which influence the utilization of obstetrical services in a Bariba region of the People's Republic of Benin, by contrasting the village of Pehunko, where customary birth practices prevail, and the administrative center of Kouande, site of the district maternity clinic, where usage of both indigenous midwives and national health services is more common.

Data on health service utilization in the People's Republic of Benin are scarce. Also lacking are clinical and analytical studies of the comprehensive role of the indigenous midwife in providing reproductive counseling and treatment, and prenatal and neonatal care, both in Benin and in West Africa in general. Such data are potentially valuable in supplementing information on beliefs and practices surrounding health-seeking behavior in Africa, and in contributing to planning of maternal and child health services which meet the actual and perceived needs of rural African populations.

The study is also intended to provide an understanding of the context for change in birth practices by demonstrating that Bariba midwifery is a therapeutic system comprising a shared set of values, beliefs and practices. Viewed from this perspective, Bariba midwifery represents one choice, currently the prevailing alternative, for obstetrical assistance. A detailed examination of the cultural context of indigenous midwifery is imperative in order to comprehend the weighing of alternative obstetrical care services, the goals and expectations of clients and practitioners, and resulting preferences. This book, then, presents a detailed clinical ethnography of Bariba birthing practices, a description of local cultural construction of obstetrical experience and behavior, and a consideration of the practical issues of integrating traditional birthing personnel and practices into the formal obstetrical delivery system.

The Bariba case is particularly interesting to consider because of the contrast between the apparent attraction of maternity services in other countries, and the reluctance to use maternity clinics and the verbal depreciation of their value by rural Bariba. It is difficult, with the inadequate statistics available, to discuss rates of utilization of maternity clinics. There does seem to be a trend towards increasing use of the Kouande clinic, although only a small percentage of district women regularly rely on its services.[1] Dispensary services, on the other hand, are more consistently utilized, especially for child care and treatment of endemic diseases. In comparison, observers elsewhere have noted that obstetrical services tend to attract clients more quickly than other services, due to the observed benefits of improved care (cf. Foster 1962, Landy 1977). Maclean, for example, found that the Yoruba held opinions on which diseases were best treated at home or at the hospital. Traditional treatment methods were held to be most relevant for treatment of the reproductive system – for impotence, sterility, and disorders of menstruation.

> . . . in the case of matters to do with reproduction, there is such a long time interval between biological cause and effect that all kinds of incidental and accidental events can appear to relate to the ultimate issue. Hence the very powerful continuing hold of traditional medicines, magical devices, prescriptions and proscriptions in this field (Maclean 1976: 309–310).

Maclean found that "empiricism triumphs in modern obstetrics" (1976:312) – that the desire for healthy offspring supplants other traditional concerns such as the objection of men to losing customary decision-making power over their wives regarding pregancy care. Maclean concludes that "the great success of hospitals in midwifery and pediatrics is generally recognized, especially among the mothers who stand to receive more immediate benefit" (314). It is intriguing, then, to consider the reasons for the slow increase in utilization of the national health obstetrical services in northern Benin.

1.2. THE SETTING

The village of Pehunko was selected as a primary research site because of its location as a crossroads market center, through which communications from surrounding villages and towns flow regularly. Because of the regular transmission of information among the populations of the settlements in this region, I hypothesized that reports concerning obstetrical care alternatives would circulate, and women would be aware of the options available to them and have some basis for evaluating the various alternatives. Moreover, from the perspective of studying a population's choice of alternative health services, Pehunko seemed appropriate due to its location at the intersection of several settlements housing maternity facilities and dispensaries. In Pehunko itself are a government nurse for curative medicine and a nurse for endemic diseases (i.e., leprosy, tuberculosis, meningitis). Pehunko, then, seemed to serve as an illustrative site to investigate the alternatives available to a Bariba woman seeking maternity care and to examine the factors involved in her choice of a midwife. An additional consideration was Pehunko's historical significance as a Bariba chiefdom, the continuing importance of Bariba traditions, and thus its utility for observing rituals and customary practices which might illuminate facets of Bariba healing.

Pehunko is located in the northwestern Atakora province; the Bariba[2] are a major ethnic group in this province, accounting for approximately 200,000 of the over 365,000 inhabitants, and occupying a wide area which stretches from the western border of Nigeria, to the eastern edge of the Atakora mountains, and from Kandi in the north to Kouande in the south (see Figure 1).

Numerous ethnic groups inhabit the Atakora, including the Somba, Yoabu, Fulbe, Dompago, Pila-Pila, and Berba. Among these, the Bariba have a lengthy history of prominence. The Bariba are patrilineal and display a decentralized social organization linking a superior provincial chief with chiefs of other provinces and with lesser chiefs. Incorporated thus in Bariba society were the ruling *wasangari* nobles, commoners (*baatombu*), slaves of varying origin, Dendi merchants, Fulbe herders, and autochthonous ethnic groups. ("Dendi" is a term long used by the French colonial administration to refer to Mande, Sarakolle, Hausa, and other Muslim settlers who were usually traders.)

Islam spread throughout the Bariba region primarily via these "Dendi" traders from Bornu and the Sudan (Lombard 1965:38). Lombard points out that whereas elsewhere in West Africa, the upper or ruling class is usually Muslim, among the Bariba, the aristocracy tended to remain animist and the subordinate Fulbe and Dendi to be Muslim. However, Islam has been gaining strength among the aristocracy of the Pehunko region. With an estimated twenty-five per cent of

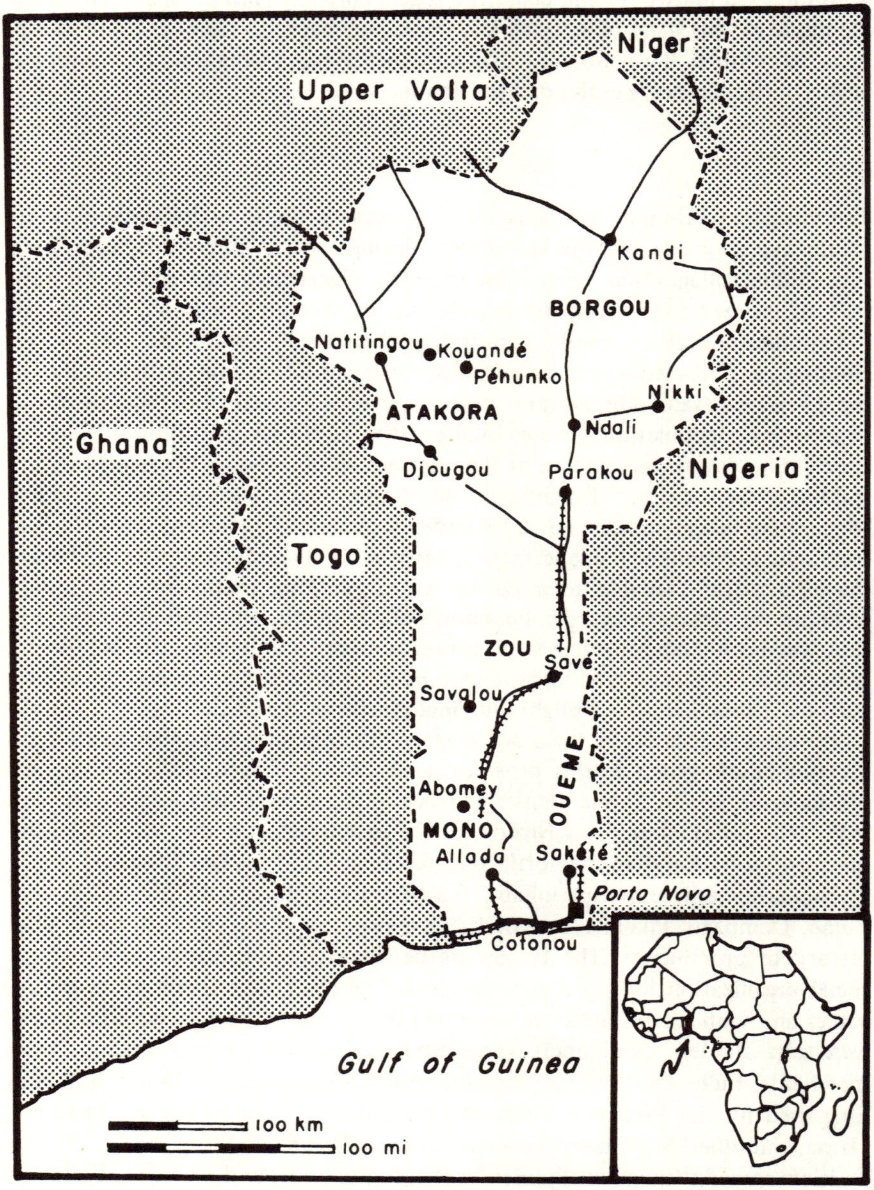

Fig. 1. Map of People's Republic of Benin.

the village population nominally Muslim, Pehunko is a stronghold of Islam in the surrounding districts.

The economy of Pehunko and of the entire region is almost completely agricultural, based on staple food crops of yams, sorghum, and millet with increasing dependence on cashcrops of peanuts, cotton, and rice. Additionally, Pehunko is an important cattle market. Currently, the name Pehunko refers both to a Commune, or agglomeration of villages, and to "Pehunko Center," the village which originally was known by that name (derivation: *Kperu*, rock; *Wonko*, black).

1.3. METHODOLOGY

The Commune of Pehunko comprised twelve villages at the time of the study (1976–77 – the District is now being reorganized). Of these village, five are Fulbe villages and were dropped from this study because of the necessity for focusing on primarily Bariba healing practices.

It quickly became apparent that political and logistical difficulties would inhibit extended interviewing of midwives and women of reproductive age in the seven Bariba villages. As a compromise measure, midwives in six villages were interviewed by means of interview schedules and informal conversations and observations over a period of a year (see Figure 2 for site locations). Of the 19 midwives interviewed, ten were selected because they had been identified as part of a government effort to find and train indigenous midwives. The others came to my attention through references from their clients or friends.

The primary difficulty in studying midwives involved arranging firsthand observations of the midwives assisting at deliveries. Because midwives resided in villages located up to 20 kilometers from Pehunko (on roads sometimes passable only on foot) where I was based, and because midwives were rarely called before a woman was in advanced labor, it was extremely difficult to arrange to be present at deliveries in villages other than those in the Pehunko center.

Constraints also deterred interviewing women of reproductive age. These constraints derived both from sampling difficulties related to recordkeeping in the Commune and to political tensions. The population of the Rural Commune of Pehunko is officially listed as 12,228 inhabitants and the population of "Pehunko Center and Neighborhoods" as 2,114, of whom 1,113 are male and 991 are female. Initially I intended to draw a random sample of women of reproductive age in Pehunko in order to determine reproductive histories, including patterns of utilization of birth attendants. However, problems arose in attempting to track down villagers listed in the census. Many names had been falsified, men were recorded as women, the dead had not been eliminated, and new family members over 14 (the eligibility age for taxes) had not been added. Thus I was obliged to abandon efforts at formal sampling based on the census.

Instead, I followed networks of my own, in both aristocratic and commoner families, expanding through the networks of those families and adding others whom I was able to find through the census reports. The number of women of reproductive age listed in the census of Pehunko Center (277) was used as the guideline for the size of the sample whom I interviewed, although I was only able to arrange interviews with 117 women (42%). These women were drawn from the six major neighborhoods of Pehunko (see Table 1).

TABLE 1
Number of women interviewed by neighborhood

Neighborhood	Estimated # women repro. age	# Women interviewed
Pehunko Center	90	66
Sinawararou	80	25
Zongo	52	17
Tance	15	6
Pehunko Gando	11	–
Gbankerou	10	9
Unknown	19	–

* (See appendix A for age breakdown of women interviewed).

Demographic data were extremely difficult to obtain on the Pehunko agglomeration. Census data were clearly not reliable and the political situation did not permit census-taking as part of the research. Since the 1972 military takeover of the national government by Mathieu Kerekou and the subsequent attempt to educate the country's population regarding the prevailing socialist philosophy, the national government has become an increasing presence in northern rural areas. Due to suspicions regarding government roles in tax collection, marketing, ideological formulation, and education, I considered a systematic effort to collect demographic data to be unfeasible. This tentative conclusion was intensified when a mercenary invasion of the country during research for the project (January 16, 1977) led to a vigorous radio broadcasting campaign to alert Beninois to be wary of speaking with or showing hospitality to foreigners, who might be mercenaries or spies. Some demographic data were obtained, nonetheless, by means of a small survey of household size. These data were obtained toward the end of the research project, by interviewing women who had participated in a survey of women of reproductive age, and gearing the questioning towards the size of the group for whom the woman cooked, washed, and so forth.

In addition to interviewing in Pehunko, I interviewed women in the village of Kouande, the district capital where the maternity clinic for the district is located. In spite of its position as district capital, Kouande was even more difficult to obtain data on than Pehunko, possibly due to political conflicts among district officials at that time. The only information which could be obtained was that the urban portion of the Commune of Kouande had an official population of 17,738; Kouande Center, where the clinic was located, had a population of about 3,100. Population figures for the rural portion of the district were unavailable and there were no available statistics on the breakdown of males and females in the district population. Thus it was not possible to accurately estimate the proportion of the district population which utilized the district clinic. Interviewing in Kouande mainly took the form of participant observation and the interviewing of women delivering at the maternity clinic over a two-month period.

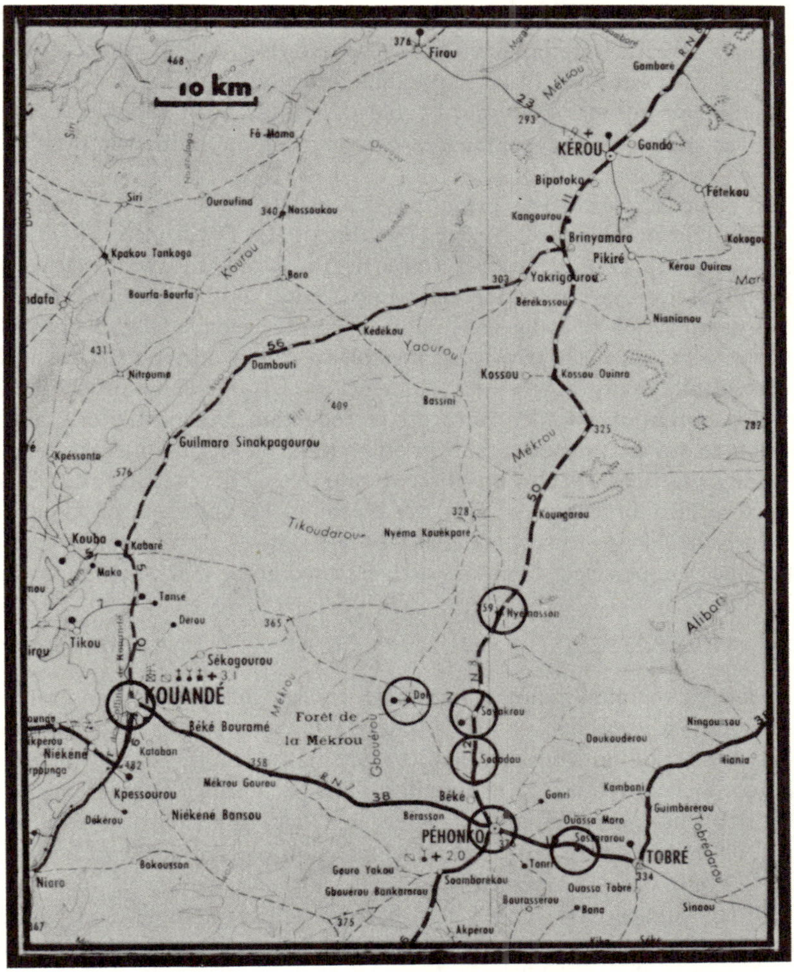

Fig. 2. Map of Site Locations.

In discussing constraints on data collection, it is also necessary to note that many customary Bariba activities such as drumming in accompaniment to rituals were restricted by the national government. Thus, traditional Bariba celebrations such as Gani (New Year), where horse races were held and tribute delivered to the chiefs, were not observed during the research period. Similarly, spirit possession cults, which rely on drumming to assist the cult members in dancing and entering a trance state, were required to obtain permission from the revolutionary council in order to meet. During most of the research, cult meetings were infrequent and/or held deep in the bush, surrounded by secrecy. This, of course, restricted observation of cult sessions and interviews with members, who were for the most part already hostile to any interest shown in their affairs and were suspicious of questioning regarding cult activities. Most data on spirit cults were obtained from two midwives, one of whom refused to directly discuss issues of ritual import but delighted in taking me to her own cult dance and to funerals so that I could watch; the other midwife was willing to answer questions and pantomime behavior for me, although she did not take me to any cult meetings.

This research project was organized as a collaboration between myself and Professor Eusèbe Alihonou, Agrégé, Director of the Department of Obstetrics and Gynecology at the National University of Benin, and was designed as a concomitant medical evaluation of maternal and child health and anthropological investigation of indigenous midwifery in the sample villages. Again, due to the political situation, it was not possible to consistently pursue the medical aspects of the study as planned. Nonetheless, Dr. Alihonou collaborated in the preparation of questionnaires on reproduction and obstetrical care and contributed to the evaluation and interpretation of various findings regarding midwifery practices. He also organized a team to conduct prenatal examinations for the women of Pehunko. This was meant to be one facet of a long-term study which did not in fact materialize; the results of the one set of consultations which are pertinent to my research are cited in the text where appropriate.

1.4. THEORETICAL PERSPECTIVES ON HEALTH CARE DECISIONS

Cross-cultural studies focusing on midwifery in general and on obstetrical care choices in particular are few, although midwifery is occasionally discussed as an illustration in considerations of alternative utilization of therapeutic options. (Mclain [1975] is one author who specifically examines this issue). More frequently, research on midwifery has been limited to descriptions of status attributes and recently, to the integration of traditional midwives into national health delivery systems.

Existing studies have tended to emphasize different topics and problems, rendering meaningful cross-cultural comparison difficult. As Jordan has noted, " . . . regarding the availability of data useful for a holistic conception of childbirth, such data are notable primarily for their absence" (Jordan 1978:5). The deficiencies of the literature derive mainly from a lack of first-hand observations of midwives in practice, which has resulted in scant data on midwifery techniques and practices.

In general, systematic research on obstetrical beliefs and practices considering birth as both a physiological and socio-cultural event is extremely limited – the best example being Jordan's *Birth in Four Cultures*, a comparative analysis of birthing systems in the United States, Holland, Sweden, and Mexico.

Because of the dearth of literature specifically devoted to the cross-cultural study of obstetrics, it is useful to consider the topic of obstetrical care choices in the general context of the utilization of alternative health care options. The analysis of health-seeking behavior where multiple health care alternatives exist has been addressed in the framework of the larger issues of culture contact, social change, and diffusion of innovations, and from the perspectives of disciplines including anthropology, sociology, and communications, among others.

As Foster and Anderson remarked in a recent work, one dominant interest in the history of medical anthropology has been the "social-aspects-of-technological change model" (Foster and Anderson 1978:vi) as exemplified by Saunders (1954), Paul (1955), Erasmus (1952) and Foster (1958, 1962). Such studies focus on the introduction of western medical services into traditional societies, and emphasize that health and disease are aspects of total culture patterns and that social factors influence health care decision. These works are more directed towards illustrating the importance of cultural and social factors in influencing technological change than in developing specific models of the process of choosing among health care alternatives.

Much of the existing research on selection of therapeutic options has relied on single-factor models. Colson classifies the generalizations and hypotheses frequently used to explain the issue of differential utilization of health services in two categories: these are "features of the disorder" as independent variables and "features of the patient" as the independent variables (Colson 1971:227). One hypothesis which falls into the category of "features of the disorder" is what Foster termed the "folk dichotomy." The essence of this hypothesis is that the use of modern as opposed to indigenous sources of therapy would correspond to the supposed origin of the disease. A disorder of natural origin would be in the domain of the modern therapist, whereas for a disorder of supernatural origin, the client would seek traditional health care (cited by Colson 1971:227).

Another set of hypotheses which Colson includes in the category of "features of the disorder" suggests that choice of a service or therapy is based on previous evidence regarding the efficacy of the alternative available. E. Fuller Torrey, for instance, suggests that behavioral disorders might most successfully be treated by indigenous practitioners whereas the outcome of treatment for somatic disorders would be more successful with modern therapy. Erasmus postulated the selection of western medical therapy to be "a matter of observed frequencies of successful outcomes" (cited by Colson, 227). Such hypotheses imply that on the basis of differential efficacy, individuals will select a particular therapeutic option, thus lending support to the idea that evaluation based on empirical observation influences the use of health services (cf. Erasmus 1952:267).

Among those hypotheses regarding "features of the patient," the most significant to mention here are the concept of relative wealth and of relative acculturation. "Relative wealth" refers to the rather evident fact that insufficient resources might inhibit prospective clients from utilizing a service; it does not, however, deal with situations where wealth is sufficient but the client nonetheless prefers not to use the service in question. From acculturation theory is derived the hypothesis that the selection of medical services depends on the degree of acculturation of the client. Colson notes the shortcomings of this approach, stating that "the basic factor ... is usually implicitly the relative degree to which one is involved in some forms of behavior that are not traditionally part of one's own culture." The problem is that "use of modern medical facilities is frequently employed as a measure of acculturation, which makes the acculturation argument tautological" (Colson 1971:228).

I intend to show that a multi-factor model is more explanatory than the models proposed by the writers mentioned above; although those models certainly contain pertinent insights into factors influencing utilization of services, they are too limited in scope. Rather, I will suggest that characteristics of the client, service, therapist and the condition interact in affecting the resulting choice. A set of salient factors, including values and beliefs, exists and may change, varying with the situation (for example, with residence of the mother or rank order of the child). The client may be viewed as weighing such factors in terms of the relative monetary and non-monetary costs. Certain combinations of factors carry differential degrees of risk, uncertainty and benefit.

The assumptions utilized derive from rational choice theory, as presented in Heath (1976) and incorporate related ideas of Rogers and Shoemaker (1971), Barth (1967, 1969), and Riley and Sermsri (1974). From the perspective of communications research, Rogers and Shoemaker (1971) attempted to integrate anthropological literature in developing an interdisciplinary model of the adoption of innovations which provides a perspective pertinent to the obstetrical choices of the Bariba.

Rogers and Shoemaker developed a model of the diffusion of innovations based on the premise that communication is essential for social change. Although this model is intended to present an interdisciplinary approach, it lacks emphasis on the effects of culture and social organization on diffusion. The diffusion of innovations model was also originally based on data from western societies, but since 1960, has been increasingly supported by research in Africa and Asia (Rogers and Shoemaker 1971:83). However, two components of the model prove useful in regarding the data on choice-making between health care alternatives. Particularly explanatory is the concept of relative advantage, which the authors subsume in a paradigm of the "innovation-decision process" under "perceived characteristics of innovations." According to Rogers and Shoemaker:

> Relative advantage is the degree to which an innovation is perceived as being better than the idea it supercedes ... Relative advantage, in one sense, indicates the intensity of the reward or punishment resulting from adoption of an innovation. There are undoubtedly a number of subdimensions of relative advantage: the degree of economic profitability, low intial cost, lower perceived risk, a decrease in discomfort, a saving in time and effort, and the immediacy of the reward (Rogers and Shoemaker 1971:139).

The authors then note that of eight investigations of the relationships between perceived attributes of innovations and their rate of adoption, almost all report a positive relationship between relative advantage and rate of adoption (139). The concept of relative advantage presupposes that the potential adopter is acting rationally, in the sense of considering the most effective means to reach a given goal – an assumption which Rogers and Shoemaker (165) make explicit; however, their concern is primarily with "objective" rationality, rather than with subjective rationality as perceived by the individual. Thus they cite Homan's measure of irrationality: "Behavior is irrational if an *outside observer* thinks that its reward is not good for a man in the long run" (165, my italics). It seems, then, that Rogers and Shoemaker are most interested in the change agent or "expert's" interpretation of rationality. They do nonetheless argue that it "is the receiver's perceptions of innovations' attributes" which affect decision-making (167).

The concept of relative advantage and more specifically of rationality in decision-making is explanatory in the Bariba example. However, relative advantage is not intended here to imply a permanent choice; that is, one choice does not necessarily supplant another, and options may be selected alternatively or simultaneously. The approach of scholars such as Rogers and Shoemaker is suggestive but not adequate. A more sophisticated approach, which focuses on choice models, is illustrated in Heath's (1976) *Rational Choice and Social Exchange*.

According to Heath, people will make decisions "rationally"; rationality here refers to the process of selecting the most effective means to reach a goal, or preferred goal where more than one goal exists. The assumption of rational choice implies (a) that although norms and roles may prescribe behavior appropriate to certain situations, people do have latitude for individual decision-making and (b) that people deliberate and weigh the advantages of options. In contrast to explanations of behavior based on unconscious drives, habitual action or societal prescription, the merit of the rational choice approach is "that it forces us to abandon the notion of man as a 'cultural dope' blindly following the norms and prescriptions of his culture. Instead it forces us to recognize man as a decision-maker who decides whether or not to conform in the light of the options available to him" (105).

In general, Health's work lends itself well to providing a model for Bariba health-seeking behavior (see also Barth 1967, for similar assumptions). The Bariba data, as will be shown, indicate that women and others involved in obstetrical decisions have a clear set of goals, that these goals are widely held among rural Bariba, and that decisions, although they may seem precipitious in any obstetrical emergency, are not capricious but measured and evaluated in terms of past experiences and current alternatives.

The analysis of alternative obstetrical care services by Bariba women is predicated upon certain assumptions which are fundamental to rational choice theory, notably that the normative approach to behavior neglects the possibility that "people usually do have choices to make, not least the choice whether to conform to the appropriate norms and role expectations. There is always some possible alternative course of action, and the costs of non-conformity are merely one set of costs to be weighed in the balance along with all the others" (Heath 1976:176).

It should be noted that one of the major criticisms of rational choice theory suggests that ordinary people are not particularly rational, that they do not weigh or evaluate alternatives as the theory postulates, that they more often choose impulsively, that they do not base decisions on complete and accurate information or try to obtain such information (Heath 1976:75). However, it is necessary to distinguish between "the rationality of a man's beliefs and knowledge and the rationality of what he does given those beliefs" (p. 76). Rational choice theory concerns the choices people make given their beliefs and is not dependent on whether people are believed to act out of self-interest, egoism, duty, friendship, or based on any particular motive. Rather, "rationality has nothing to do with the goals which men pursue but only with the means they use to achieve them" (Heath 1976:79).

It is certainly true that complete information may not be available to or utilized by individuals. In addition, constraints of which decision-makers are not aware (for example, class factors, national policies, international economic competition) may impinge on choices made. Nonetheless, it seems desirable to differentiate the issues of social forces impinging on individuals (and beyond their domain of awareness) and the decision-making process in which the individual believes herself/himself to be engaged. That is, people operate on the premise that they do have choices to make, and that they have bases upon which to make decisions. That they may be unaware of all factors comprehensible to an external analyst does not negate the validity of studying the choice-making process given the facts, beliefs, and values in relation to which the individual acts.

Correspondingly, Ortiz states that "rationality of behavior does not imply that there is a constant conscious awareness of having made a choice or even the ability to express it verbally in terms of quantities or factors (Ortiz 1967: 196). It is important to note, though, that the number of alternatives available to an individual depends on the information available to that individual or significant others (Prattis 1973:48; Ortiz 1967:220). In the Bariba context, access to information to a certain extent correlates with social class; thus civil servants and those employed by government agencies or Europeans have greater access to reports about health services, quality of care, procedures for utilization, and so forth. Town-dwellers also have greater access to information than villagers residing off the main roads, due to rumor networks via shops, market communication, politicization of health care, and resultant attempts at publicizing and advocating use of national health care clinics. After more than 25 years of existence, it is the rare individual who is unaware of the existence of maternity clinics and of their function. Nonetheless, those who are involved in "modern" occupations, particularly the civil service sector (including the agricultural service), and who reside in administrative centers have much more constant and fuller access to information regarding health care alternatives. This differential access to information affects selection of an obstetrical service: although everyone may be aware of the actual existence of the alternatives, certain sectors of the population are better informed than others as to such aspects of the clinic alternative as expected behavior for a patient, familiarity with bureaucratic procedures, and, probably, treatment procedures and staff behavior.

Overall, in the Bariba case, the data suggest that people minimize costs and try to assure reaching their goal to the extent that these two attempts can be attained simultaneously. The probable goals of Bariba women seeking a delivery setting are listed below. These goals are intended to represent the client perspective, taking as ideal types a farmer's wife in the village of Pehunko and a trader's wife in the administrative center of Kouande, where the maternity clinic is located. The goals are listed roughly in order of priority:

Farmer's Wife: Home Delivery	Trader's Wife: Clinic Delivery
live mother and baby	live mother and baby
live mother	live mother
live baby	live baby
witchcraft control	aspirations to upward mobility
manifestation of high standards of female behavior	prestige associated with "civil servant" behavior
minimize costs (infrastructural)	minimize costs (infrastructural)

These goals can be understood in terms of "strategy," where "strategy" refers to selecting a means of meeting goals. Selecting a particular delivery setting and type of birth assistant has implications for the goals which are most likely to be met – for example, witchcraft control is unlikely to be assured in a national health maternity clinic. The preferred strategy seems to be to attempt to meet the entire set of goals if possible. However, as suggested previously, in situations such as obstetrical emergencies, people may adopt the strategy of preserving as many goals as possible. Thus the goals of witchcraft control and high standards of female behavior may be sacrificed in order to assure "live mother" if the life of the mother appears at risk.

A necessary consideration in the study of decision-making is the identification of decision-makers, including the differential influence of individuals based on gender, age, and other status attributes. In this regard, Janzen's (1978) work on the choice of therapeutic alternatives among the Bakongo in lower Zaire is suggestive, especially because research on health care decisions in sub-Saharan Africa is scant. Janzen organized his study around what he referred to as the therapy managing group, primarily composed of kin in the rural areas, and additionally, of work and church associates in the urban context. According to Janzen, western and traditional medical systems are complementary in course of therapy, but irreconcilably disparate in terms of cultural logic. Each system possesses an internal rationale, linking therapeutic technique to symptoms or problem identification. These disparate systems are often utilized in conjunction with one another to terminate a case satisfactorily via referral among/between the kin therapy management group, African healers, African personnel working in the European system, and European physicians (to a lesser extent).

According to Janzen, the Bakongo have a clear concept of the focus and limits of western medicine, and delineate it as a separate therapeutic system, effective, but for a narrow range of purposes. The primary deficiency of western therapy seems to be its inability to deal with problems of wider social etiology. Choice of a therapy then becomes dependent on the therapy management group's diagnosis of the problem.

One of Janzen's most interesting suggestions is that in a decision-making process, there may be majority/minority decisions within the kin group. The majority decision may be to consult a diviner, the minority to consult a physician. If the first decision proves unsatisfactory or only partially resolves the problem, the minority decision may increase to first priority. This process will be shown to occur also with decisions regarding obstetrical care among Bariba women.

Two significant differences are evident between the situation among the Bakongo and that of Bariba women. According to Janzen, the Bakongo deal with the discrepancies between medical systems by utilizing indigenous healers to treat the issues of wider social etiology of illness, while utilizing western therapy for obtaining medicines to relieve physical symptoms. For example Janzen states that "when a disease is diagnosed as having a social or mystical cause, the therapeutic tradition prescribes simultaneous treatment for localized symptoms and wider causes": (191). This dichotomy has been suggested for other African societies as well (cf. Maclean 1976; Frankenberg and Leeson 1976; Asuni 1979). In the case of Bariba obstetrics, however, it is not as feasible to utilize a maternity clinic or hospital for a delivery and simultaneously to use indigenous healers to deal with significant issues of etiology which are not perceived as considerations by western medical personnel.

A second difference between the Bakongo and Bariba contexts is that the complexity of the therapy management group appears to be much greater (more formal and with greater participation) among the Bakongo than in the situation where Bariba are deciding how to deal with a delivery. Among the Bakongo, the decision-making responsibility is often assumed by matrilineal kin ranging from mother (biological or classificatory) to mother's brothers and siblings (130). Spouses do not usually have an especially significant voice in the proceedings and sufferers "retain decision-making rights only if they are adult, usually male, capable of walking and travelling, and financially able to pay for care" (130). In contrast, Bariba obstetrical care decisions primarily involve the patient and the women of the household holding position of greatest authority (e.g., mother-in-law, father's sister, father's mother). Rarely are group discussions held either formally or informally.

Analysis of the Bariba data will include a consideration of the rewards and costs of obstetrical care alternatives to different sectors of the population. In determining the perceived costs of the alternatives, two factors will be emphasized. These are (1) the extent to which homophily/heterophily of therapists and clients affecting decisions and (2) the cultural meaning of efficacy in affecting decisions.[3] The homophily/heterophily dichotomy is one which was set forth by Rogers and Shoemaker in discussing opinion leadership and its effect on the process of diffusion of innovations. In this context, homophily is defined as "the degree to which pairs of individuals who interact are similar in certain attributes such as beliefs, values, education, social status and the like," (210) whereas heterophily refers to the "degree to which pairs of individuals who interact are different in certain attributes" (210). Rogers and Shoemaker hypothesize that "change agent success is positively related to . . . homophily with clients" (242).

This proposition in conjunction with the comparative literature cited above led to the pre-fieldwork formation of a hypothesis: most village women, other than wives of upwardly mobile men, would prefer to utilize the services of indigenous midwives rather than nurse-midwives. The reason for this preference was suggested to be the lack of role congruency between the position of nurse-midwife and indigenous midwife and correspondingly, the lack of fulfillment by nurse-midwives of role expectations held by rural clients. The discrepancy in attributes between client and nurse-midwife parallels that between indigenous midwife and nurse-midwife. This explanation was found to be relevant in contributing to the understanding of preferences for birth assistance. The implications of this finding for the rational choice approach are that one primary consideration in the selection of a birth assistant is "can the midwife/healer accomplish the task at hand?" Whether a particular type of healer will be selected by clients depends on attributes of the person who could successfully achieve the desired goals; the question of successfully accomplishing healing responsibilities, then, incorporates expectations about the attributes of the role occupant, such as sociological and career characteristics. In order to fullfill role expectations, then, the indigenous midwife must demonstrate attributes which fall within an acceptable range to the client population, rendering her reasonably homophilous.

Similarity in attributes such as beliefs, values, past experience with health care practices, influence prospective clients in their selection among health care alternatives. Thus a client will tend to prefer the practitioner who is "homophilous" and shares the above attributes and expectations regarding roles of patients and healers. Correspondingly, the absence of homophily as manifest in the relationship between most rural Bariba women and clinic nurse-midwives operates as a constraint on prospective clients evaluating the possibility of utilizing a maternity clinic. In subsequent chapters, an attempt will be made to show that indigenous midwives and their clients are homophilous, that the majority of prospective clients and nurse-midwives are not homophilous, and that lack of homophily renders the maternity clinic option less desirable than home delivery to the rural population.

The second issue, the cultural meaning of efficacy, is significant because of the basic assumption that when choosing a health care service or assistant, people seek a type of assistance which they believe will "work" to solve the problem, however that problem is defined. Kleinman has addressed this issue in his discussion of the cultural construction of clinical reality, where he suggests that "patient-doctor interactions are transactions between explanatory models, transactions often involving major discrepancies in cognitive content as well as therapeutic values, expectations and goals" (Kleinman 1978a:254). The decision of prospective patients to select a particular therapeutic option will in part depend on the degree to which patient and practitioner share models of clinical reality. Similarly in evaluating a health service, Donabedian urges that the criterion of "shared definition" is of first-order significance.

> Because illness, and particularly 'health' are to varying degrees socially, rather than technically, defined, that organization is best that has mechanisms for the inclusion of client and social perspectives on 'health' and illness . . . " (Donabedian 1972:105)

Where a shared definition of health and illness is absent, then, a service cannot offer health care which addresses adequately the perceived needs of the population; such a service will predictably not be a preferred choice among a majority of the client population.

In this research, the problem at hand is the Bariba definition of pregnancy and birth in contrast to that held implicit by cosmopolitan clinic personnel. Critical to the definition is the variable meaning of the concept of "work" or efficacy; the Bariba data indicate that the cultural definition of the meaning of birth in relation to both cosmological and social factors greatly influences the preference for one sort of birth assistant. This topic will be developed, following an explanation of relevant aspects of Bariba culture, with particular reference to witchcraft beliefs.

In subsequent chapters, hypotheses regarding obstetrical care decision-making will be considered. These hypotheses will be examined in light of the Bariba data but have implications wider than this delimited context. The hypotheses under consideration fall into several major categories:

Assumptions Underlying the Model of Health Service Utilization

(1) People usually do have choices to make; they have given wants and values and will select the most effective means to reach a goal or set of goals.

(2) A primary consideration affecting a decision will be comparative costs

of alternatives; these costs may be conceptualized as both monetary and non-monetary costs.

Features of the Model

(1) A multi-factor model of utilization of health care services is more explanatory than single-factor models previously devised by other analysts of health service utilization.

Features of Clients Seeking Obstetrical Care

(1) Social characteristics such as education and occupation are related to preferences for obstetrical assistance and setting; thus most rural women, other than wives of civil servants[4] and wealthy traders will prefer home deliveries except in obstetrical emergencies believed to surpass the competence of indigenous midwives.

Features of Practitioners

(1) Clients will select a practitioner based on the degree of homophily (similarity in attributes) between themselves and the practitioner. Absence of homophily is considered to operate as a constraint to clients evaluating the desirability of alternative obstetrical assistance.

(2) Choices of practitioner, moreover, will be related to expectations held by clients regarding attributes, techniques, and practices characteristic of a competent midwife.

Features of the Disorder

(1) Clients will select a practitioner or service on the basis of the definition of the problem to be treated and correspondingly, on the basis of decisions regarding the type of practitioner most competent to deal with the disorder as diagnosed.

(2) Where a shared definition of the problem is absent, a service cannot offer care addressing the perceived needs of the population and will not be a preferred choice to a majority of the population.

Features of the Decision-Making Process

(1) The domain of reproduction represents one of the primary arenas in which women control decision-making.

(2) Women's decisions regarding choices of obstetrical assistance are not precipitous but are the outcome of cultural expectations, past experiences and existing alternatives.

Chapters 2 and 3 will present the cultural context of therapeutic choice and a description of beliefs and practices surrounding reproductive processes;

Chapter 4 will examine features of the decision-making process, in particular, women's control of the domain of reproduction;

Chapter 5 focuses on implications of role expectations for birth assistance and assesses hypotheses regarding features of the practitioner;

Chapter 6 examines features of the disorder – detailing the definition of birth as an event and consequences for obstetrical care choices;

Chapter 7 and 8 comprise case studies; and

Chapter 9 includes further discussion of features of clients and practitioners in the national health service setting. This chapter also presents a concluding discussion of the rationality of health care decision-making.

In general, the present study of the factors influencing use of alternative obstetrical assistance is set in a presentation of the social context for decision-making. The discussion of social environment in this Bariba region will focus particularly on the interrelationship between religion, morality, and healing, and include aspects of stratification and the role of women in Bariba society. Moreover, beliefs and practices surrounding reproductive processes will be detailed. A significant point which the presentation of these data is intended to support is that although decisions may appear to be impulsive or precipitous, especially in an obstetrical crisis, such decisions are based on previously acquired models of appropriate behavior. The moment of decision-making, then, represents a point in time but more accurately reflects a process comprising a range of cultural expectations and past experiences in which context current alternatives are evaluated and selected.

CHAPTER 2

THE CULTURAL CONTEXT OF THERAPEUTIC CHOICE

The intent of the following chapter is to present data on religion, cosmology and concepts of morality among the Bariba that will serve as a foundation for explaining the bases of therapeutic choices made by Bariba women. The central hypothesis of the chapter is that decisions regarding the utilization of alternative medical services are largely derived from the diagnosis of the sickness or disorder that is presenting a problem to the sufferer and significant others. Thus, the logic of therapeutic choice must relate problem identification to therapy techniques and specialists' roles – only then do actions taken in response to sickness begin to make sense (Janzen 1978:127). The determination of a diagnosis is necessarily related to beliefs and assumptions regarding sickness causation; as Maclean noted "treatment is always related to explanation since, in the absence of some idea of causation, the response to symptoms is arbitrary or irrational" (Maclean 1976:290). This chapter then, seeks to discuss Bariba concepts of causation of sickness in the broader context of beliefs regarding the causes of misfortune, assumptions regarding human nature, and conceptions of a "general order of existence" (cf. Geertz 1966:8–12) in Bariba culture. In general, the chapter will attempt to sketch the range of beliefs, values and expectations that comprise major assumptions upon which therapeutic choices are based.

2.1. BARIBA CONCEPTIONS OF THE ORDER OF THE UNIVERSE

The patterned set of ideas and practices regarding sickness which comprises the Bariba medical system is best illuminated in the context of the Bariba understanding of the nature of the universe and man's relationship to that universe. Ideas and assumptions concerning sickness and attempts to deal with sickness will be seen to represent a subset of the larger system of beliefs regarding reality, both empirically and unempirically verifiable (cf. Van Baal 1971:3). In this regard, Pellegrino suggested that "medicine is an exquisitely sensitive indicator of the dominant cultural characteristics of any era, for man's behavior before the threats and realities of illness is necessarily rooted in the conception he has constructed of himself and his universe" (Pellegrino quoted in Foster 1978: 39).

Bariba ideas of disease causation are rooted in concepts of the nature of the universe. This universe is presided over by *gusunɔ̃*, the creator of man and commander of death. The word *gusunɔ̃* also encompasses the sky, stars, and clouds (*gusunɔ̃ wɔllɔ*: God on high). Some say that this is because *gusunɔ̃* is on the other side of the sky and that God is everywhere. Although the name of *gusunɔ̃* is invoked frequently in pious comfort ("God Is,") in interjections ("By God!") and as the causative agent in misfortunes and blessings, in a practical sense, the various spirits receive more attention and are more specifically detailed in nature than is *gusunɔ̃*.[5]

The generic term for spirit is *bun* (pl. *bunu*); spirits often reside in rocks, trees and animals. The village of Pehunko, for example, is named after certain black rocks which contain the patron spirits of the village (although some elderly villagers say that since the Revolution, the *bunu* have left the rocks). One Bariba commoner family is held responsible for sacrifices to these spirits; in the event of a village-wide catastrophe such as an epidemic of measles or meningitis, the rocks will cry out. When the rocks cry, the family member responsible will check with the chief, arrange a consultation with the spirits to communicate with them and learn what misfortune is about to strike. If the rocks are heard and a sacrifice is made, the misfortune will be less severe. In sacrificing to the spirits in the rocks, the sacrifice may also be offered to God simultaneously (thus it is said "God has the sacrifice") but it is the spirits who are of true importance.

Spirits may similarly reside in animals; the patron spirits of the village of Doh, for instance, are a three-generation family of crocodiles. These spirits used to appear on Fridays and Sundays but left Doh in a fit of pique when certain taboos were transgressed (women washed pepper spoons in the swamp and also their menstrual rags) and moved to the village of Tikou where the people are more well-behaved. Spirits, whether residing in animals, rocks or trees are addressed by men and urged to intercede with God. Not all spirits are so benevolent, however. Spirits of the bush, such as *wereku* or *zini* exist and cause sickness or madness if seen by human eyes. *Zini*, who are white and are so tall that their heads are in the sky, are particularly dreaded. They live in trees and their unique quality is the capacity to transform themselves into people or animals and delude humans. Stories abound of men who become transfixed by a beautiful girl who lures them to a graveyard where she suddenly is transformed into her true self – a *zini*. The person then falls gravely ill or dies. Only a powerful person dares to attack a *zini*, at which time it may turn into a rabbit and run away. *Wereku*, on the other hand, are tiny people with huge bushy heads of hair and their feet on backwards who also cause madness or sickness but may also be inhabited by spirits which in turn possess humans. Both *wereku* and *zini* represent a distinction between "bush" and "village," or organization and chaos and are greatly feared.

A multitude of spirits exist who may possess humans; they are generally known as *bunu* but also have special names, depending on their characteristics. Such spirits are not usually harmful to people unless they come to "sit on the head of someone" and the family refuses to accept them. In such situations, they will cause sickness and possibly death. In contrast to the spirits of animals, rocks, trees mentioned above, those spirits which possess people do not intercede with God on behalf of humans; the presence of possession spirits is manifest only during a possession state.

Like some spirits, the dead (*gɔribu*) can be requested to intercede with God on behalf of their descendants. Most often, though, the dead are not contacted unless the deceased made a deathbed statement indicating that the death was not a "natural" one. In such a case, the dying person may request the family to contact him/her on a certain date at which time the sorcerer will be named or revenge planned, or they may ask who was responsible for the death. To contact the dead, the living require the services of a specialist known as a *bunkɔsɔ*, who communicates with the dead or with the dead or with spirits from a special house designed for that purpose. Not every village has a communicator currently and even in the past it seems that the *bunkɔsɔ* served a region. Pehunko has no *bunkɔsɔ*.

One well-known case of the revenge of the dead involved a woman who died near Pehunko. Before her death, she asked for a Bariba burial but her brothers, who had converted to Islam, buried her in a Muslim ceremony. Shortly after the burial, her daughter was stricken with abcesses all over her body which no treatment seemed to cure. Eventually a *bunkɔsɔ* was consulted and contacted the dead mother, who expressed her dissatisfaction with the burial. After the corpse was disenterred and reburied in the desired ceremony, the abcesses disappeared. Rarely, the dead may be contacted in order to obtain information; for example, one daughter asked her dead mother "why do I have a hard life" and her mother said that "life is transient . . . " The dead themselves may harm either strangers or members of the family if they were forced to die an unnatural death (teenage, murder, poison, etc.). But in general, it is the living who are suspected first in cases of misfortune, including sickness.

The attribution of responsibility for sickness causation is based on the Bariba conception of the universe as composed of opposing forces (chaos-order; abnormality-normality; evil-good) and of objects which contain forces (rocks, trees, animals). Man, then, attempts to manipulate these forces to his advantage. A basic assumption is that human nature is intrinsically evil and that people, motivated by ill-will, will attempt to manipulate the "powers of nature" to their own advantage by using these powers against others. Man, then, is potentially dangerous and is expected to attempt to dissipate or reduce the powers of others, hence reducing their chances of assuring a rich life. Thus proverbs advise:

> Flee Man and Sit in the Sun
> The Tongue of Man is Evil
> Man is Difficult

In general, the distinction between natural and supernatural seems ambiguous in Bariba thinking; there are few "natural" causes of sickness and/or death other than death apparently due to very old age, for which the Bariba say "*u tura*: " . . . he arrived."

The classic Bariba response to questioning regarding the frequency of allegations of "poisoning" (sorcery) is to bemoan the ill will of others and to cite the proverb "As long as there is betrayal, there will be poison" (*dukiri kun kpa dobonu kun daa gare*). "*Dukiri*," loosely translated as betrayal, or sometimes treason, refers to situations involving love, money, vengeance, shame. "*Dukiri*" according to one old lady usually refers to a situation where someone makes you unhappy by ignoring expectations. Thus a man works for several years to win a wife, helping the woman's father in the fields and bringing gifts and suddenly the woman marries someone else. This is *dukiri* and the aggrieved man will seek revenge. When co-wives steal each others' menstrual rags to use in sorcery against each other, it is because one wife feels that the husband has preferred the other. In one case in the village of Yemasson, a midwife claimed that she had been poisoned (as manifest by a swelling in her stomach like a pregnancy) when she helped a pregnant woman who was unable to deliver due to the interference of "an enemy." When the midwife Bouko successfully aided the woman, the enemy, thwarted by Bouko, attacked her instead. This is also *dukiri*.

One old person specified that times have changed – people now poison one another for riches or because another has many children and they have none, but this is not *dukiri*, it is jealousy (*tusira*). Although it is likely that in the past as well as currently, people poisoned from jealousy as well as from a sense of betrayal, it seems clear that whichever emotion is at the root of the actions, Bariba are wary of the motivations of others and expect harm from both the human and spirit worlds. Such expectations result in careful attention to protective amulets, jewelry, medicines, and overall, to secrecy in dealings external to the household or with close relatives of household members in other villages.

The alleged goal of the Bariba who seeks to diminish the powers of his fellow Bariba is to render others weak, helpless, and poor. An example of the state in which one Bariba might like to see another came to light when I traveled to a small village with a young woman who intended to visit her relatives there. We walked through a deserted compound, belonging to her uncle. Although it was noon, no one was about; no fires were lit, no cooking underway, and all doors were shut. The young woman explained that several years ago, that same compound had been bustling with women and children but due to conflicts among co-wives, illnesses and deaths, and a fire, only two adult men were left, with no one to cook for them. "This is the way 'they' like people to be," the woman said, "with an empty house and no cooking fires." "They," representing significant others motivated by ill-will and aspirations to augment their own benefits, were deemed responsible for the sad state of the uncle's household. Implied in this sequence is the idea that for one person to be successful in life, others must suffer and their wealth – whether cattle, children, wives, or anything equated with *dam*, or power – must be diminished. One means of weakening others is to cause them to be afflicted with sickness, often by using substances such as roots, leaves, herbs, animal parts, to be ingested; or poisoned objects which are buried; property of the victim which will be infused with harmful power by the assailant and lead to sickness if counter-measures are not undertaken, and so forth.

Sickness, however, is not always or solely caused by human intervention and it is in this sense that the natural and supernatural, or the human and suprahuman merge. Even in the case of a death known to be due to poisoning by another individual, it is said that the hour of death is fixed by God and "he whom God has called is the one whom the poisoner kills." Sicknesses can be caused by man, witches, sorcerers, ancestors, spirits, or contact with objects or breach of taboos which carry the penalty of affliction. Whatever the category of cause, the power of the forces of the universe is involved, whether in the form of willful human intervention by manipulation of powers in substances (sorcery); uncontrollable, inherent power (witchcraft); or powers of the spirit world which includes ancestors, spirits, and God.

In a discussion of the ontological status of medicine, Glick conceptualized illness as a subset of the domain of religious ideas linked via the element of "power," "power existing as a manifest attribute of persons and of objects in their environment" (Glick 1967:33). This proposition corresponds closely both with the Bariba conceptualization and an etic interpretation of the Bariba belief system. Glick then asks "who or what is powerful in this society," how is this power controlled," and "what is mobilized to serve human purposes?" (Glick 1967:34)

I have already noted that two broad spectrums of power formerly existed in Bariba society, and continued to exist, although weakened by the colonial presence and national government until 1972. These were the secular, political and non-secular domains of power. Within the non-secular domain were healers, diviners, clairvoyants, spirit cult members, sorcerers and witches, to mention the most noteworthy. Although it is the implicit goal of every Bariba to increase his power in this domain, few succeed. Those who do are primarily elderly males; power increases with age (as well as knowledge and experimentation, which may also correspond to age). Some few elderly women may also become powerful.

To what does "power" refer in this sense? As Glick defined it, power refers to an attribute of persons and of objects (33). More specifically, this power may exist as knowledge; as a capacity to transcend the human world and comm-nicate with spirits; as an ability to read the future; as a strength of character which acts as a bulwark for an individual against external forces. An individual may, for example, manifest his power by facing a *zini* and rather than fleeing, hitting it with a staff to transform it into a rabbit. Another may possess potent medicines to heal, while yet another may be responsible for communicating with the patron spirits of the village. Those whose primary intent is to do evil form a special category. This includes witches, who are believed to be sent by God, and manifest themselves at birth (witchcraft cannot be transmitted by blood or milk, in contrast to the neighboring Gourmanche and Djerma), and sorcerers. Those sorcerers who utilize poison made from corpses are particularly dreaded. Witches harm only their patrilineal kin, as opposed to sorcerers who mainly choose non-family members as their victims; an exception to this rule is that during inheritance disputes, kin may attempt to use sorcery against one another. However, the power which enables one to do good can also be turned to evil, depending on the motivation of the individual, thus all power represents ambiguity. According to prevalent Bariba belief, men are endlessly engaged in a struggle to manipulate the forces of nature to maintain a precarious balance of good/order/normality and to concomitantly achieve their own individual ends; the strength or power which men acquire may be put to beneficial purposes or may be used malevolently, subject to the baseness of human desires but all use of power by humans is mediated by the spirit world.

2.2. DIAGNOSIS AND TREATMENT

With reference to healing, diagnosis "involves ideas about sources of disease-causing power and treatment involves attempts to overcome that power" (Glick 1967:34). The symbolism of fighting and trying to overcome the power of the disease is evident in an expression used when the death of someone who has had a long illness is announced – "*u kpanna*," he wasn't able (to overcome it).

A distinction might be made between illnesses or sickness, and ailments (Glick 1967:39). Ailments are defined by Glick as "relatively minor and temporary afflictions lacking significant socio-cultural antecedents or consequences" (39) and these conditions he relegates to a separate category of experience, in contrast to illnesses "which have named socio-culturally relevant causes and require culturally defined and socially mediated responses" (39). The Bariba data suggest that it is the elements of time and gravity of the disorder which determine whether a condition is, to use Glick's terminology, a mere ailment or an illness. That is, any ailment may after a certain time period, be identified as an illness. Thus an ailment (such as sprains, minor burns, skin ulcers, infected insect bites) which Bariba consider a "natural" disorder, carries the potential for progressing to an illness, or "unnatural" disorder, whether by misdiagnosis of the original affliction, or evolution of the condition (cf. Maclean 1976:289).

The Bariba diagnose primarily on the basis of symptom presentation or type of death. Figure 3 presents some examples of diagnostic criteria.

Spirits are rarely the cause of death and only occasionally of illness; their major function is to intervene with God on behalf of man. Illnesses of type (2) may be evidence that the victim has committed some wrong-doing; for example, certain treated substances (*waaburu*) may be placed in a field to protect against thieves. The thief who enters such a field will manifest symptoms such as a black pimple eruption or swelling thus indicating his contact with the treated substance.

Obstetrical complications will be elaborated in subsequent chapters. Here, however, it is necessary to state that obstetrical complications fit generally into the pattern of beliefs and practices regarding sickness with the exception that intrinsically, pregnancy and delivery are not considered pathological processes. Rather, pregnancy is a normal physiological process, and complaints of pregnancy do not usually require divination or discussions of ultimate causation. However, should a complication occur, it is then defined as a pathological process and

Symptoms	Ultimate cause	Remedial action
1. swelling* sudden death death by violence (e.g., lightening)	suspect sorcery	family of victim consults a diviner privately
2. swelling swollen throat black pimple eruption madness	sorcery (victim rightfully being punished for crime)	family or victim consults diviner privately
3. madness faintness cold body shallow, rapid breathing difficulty in breathing	sorcery, witchcraft spirit possession witchcraft witchcraft	private divination may be followed by cult initiation
4. "rotting vagina"	sorcery	private divination
5. lingering illness	sorcery	private divination
6. lingering illness of elderly	old age, God	no divination unless dying person requrests
7. death of neonates and small children	God, spirit world	usually no divination
8. epidemic	spirit world	public divination on behalf of villages
9. abnormalities of labor and delivery	witchcraft; occasionally sorcery or breach of taboo	usually no divination except for repeated OB deaths in a family

* Death by "swelling" (snakebite, for instance) is particularly abhorrent to Bariba; it is said that no one should inherit from a person who dies in this state. Thus his goods will be destroyed and not divided. When a person is bitten by a snake, in order to avoid this curse, his/her head is shaven as a purification, but this may not be sufficient to ward off death or to allow inheritance. The connection between swelling, snakebite and an "unclean death" seems evident, but unclear. Snakebite may indicate witchcraft; thus some advocate killing the snake, checking it to see if it has intestines, because a snake without intestines is clearly supernatural. Perhaps the horror of the swelling is linked to witchcraft. Death due to witchcraft but manifest in other presentations, such as during labor, is also greatly dreaded.

Fig. 3. Concepts of Sickness Causation among Bariba.

dealt with accordingly, within the general context of Bariba sickness concepts and beliefs regarding causation of misfortune. This issue will be discussed in detail in subsequent chapters. However, one complication, *tigpiru*, is worthy of some discussion at this point because it is such a common complaint of both pregnant and non-pregnant Bariba.

Tigpiru is a condition that afflicts both men and women but is most prevalent among married women, especially pregnant women. The term *tigpiru* refers to a condition characterized by lower abdominal pain or back pain. Intrinsically it is considered to be an internal growth which, as the illness progresses, becomes red, takes a round form "like an egg," and protrudes through the anus or the vagina. If the illness does not protrude, it may lie flat in the abdomen and cause swollen legs and feet. *Tigpiru* is usually considered a "natural" disorder, likely to afflict women and perhaps men, and home remedies and specialists' cures abound to treat the condition. However, *tigpiru* can also inhibit labor and delivery and in such cases, witchcraft may be suspected.

In general, obstetrical complications are attributed to adultery, in which case the woman must confess and call out the true name of the father or the child will refuse to be born; sometimes to breach of taboo; or to witchcraft by the unborn child. Occasionally, sorcery may be the cause, but no such instances came to my attention and Bariba claim they are rare. Witchcraft appears to be the most likely explanation for a maternal death, fetal abnormalities or other severe complications. It is interesting, however, that although infant witches are a common subject of conversation among Bariba, there is little mention of adult witches; sorcery, or deliberate malevolence by adults is a subject of more frequent comment.

Sorcery may be indicated by various symptoms and/or types of condition; for example, the abrupt onslaught of a disorder may signal sorcery, as when a child awakens screaming in the night and dies soon after. Because sickness is so frequently attributed to sorcery, two suspected cases will be described. In the first case, a 21-year-old woman, married and mother of a 15-month-old child, awakened on market day and began to prepare food to sell at the market. Feeling abdominal cramps, she went to the fields to relieve herself but was unable to walk back; she eventually crawled to a house where the women tried to feed her porridge, but she vomited. Finally, the women carried her home. The women of her own household asked her what she had eaten or drunk but she claimed that she hadn't taken anything. They treated her briefly, and decided she was better. Then she complained of pains in her legs, so the women told the household children to massage her legs while they went to market. When they returned in the afternoon, she was dead. Because of the mysterious onslaught of sickness and her precipitous death, sorcery was suspected (although some women claimed she had tried to abort and had poisoned herself). Her father, the son of the former village chief, was convinced that someone was trying to harm him through his child; the woman's mother, who had only that one living child, was certain that someone meant to harm her. The young woman was buried inside the walls of the courtyard in order to prevent the sorcerer from dancing on her grave, thus rendering himself invisible and undentifiable. The mother consulted a diviner but the family claimed that a definite result was not forthcoming.

In a second case, as I was walking down a major road of Pehunko, I heard sudden shriekings and wailing and saw a woman in a household bordering the road, tearing her hair, and others coming outside. This was the household of the high Muslim priest, Baalimam, and eventually it became clear that one of his wives had just died. After several days, the story could be pieced together. The wife had gone to a funeral two days before her death. While at the funeral, she had suddenly felt dizzy and fainted. Neighbors carried her home and Baalimam called several old men to come and burn medicines (*duku*) to bring the woman's soul back to her body. Sorcery was already suspected (perhaps especially because Baalimam was, even in the post-revolutionary period, a powerful man, said to have "unclean hands" himself, and would be a likely candidate for an attack). When she awakened, the woman had a headache so the next day she went to the dispensary where she was given aspirin. Shortly thereafter, her menstrual period ceased prematurely; her body became colder and colder, and she died. Some speculated that the aspirin had caused her death but most agreed that the fainting and cold body were clear indicators that someone had deliberately stolen her soul. Although divination was employed to determine the cause of death and the evil-doer, again, in this case, the sequel to the divination was not made public and the family claimed that investigation would be pursued.

Breach of taboo was also mentioned as a possible cause of sickness. The symptoms presented may depend, in this type of causation, on the particular taboo – for example, a person who eats salt after a delivery, when it is forbidden, will go blind. Neglect of obligations may also cause affliction or even death. In one actual case, a man died of snakebite, which in this case was blamed on the victim's refusal to go to the assistance of a sick brother and sister in the preceding weeks.

In sum, sickness may be provoked by various causes; as one elderly blind woman said regarding the loss of eyesight – it might have come from God, man, or witches, or in the words of another, sickness is in the air, in the bush, and all around us. Objects, whether animate or inanimate, may cause sickness when they have been "charged" with power by a human. Thus, one rather difficult to classify sickness allegedly caused by an object is "*ampoule*." "*Ampoule*" is a word meaning "light bulb" in French. *Ampoule* was described by the healer who specializes in treating this condition as a sickness of coughing, paleness and thinness. According to the healer, "from the beginning of the world" there has been *ampoule*; but others claim it is caused by people shining a flashlight directly on a person. Yet others say the sickness is called *ampoule* because the treatment is cupping and when the victim is cupped, the disease is removed and it looks white like a light bulb.

Some Bariba claim that all diseases are caused by man or by the dead who are irked by a lack of respect or breach of taboo. In the event of breach of taboo, a spirit will come in a dream during the night, suck the blood of the victim and sickness will follow, usually with vague symptoms such as diffuse pain, feeble body, or impotence. A diviner will usually be consulted. However, although some claim that man, by his manipulations, is at the root of all sickness, diseases exist which seem to be beyond human control and fit purely in the domain of the spirit world. Two such sicknesses are "squirrel" (*saagu, wirugu*) and "rabbit" (*gbigbiku*), both of which are caused by contact with the animals in question. In the case of "squirrel," a pregnant women is affected by this condition when she throws food scraps away in a field and a squirrel gets them; her child will later be stricken with fallen fontanel ("split head.") This condition, then, is not caused by an enemy, although one might argue that the woman's own negligence is at fault. "Rabbit" is caused by the fright a pregnant woman suffers when a rabbit crosses her path; she may also be affected if she walks in the urine of a rabbit (albeit unknowingly) or if a rabbit enters the courtyard at night to eat scraps and it howls . . . subsequently, the sickness manifests itself in the young child. "Rabbit" seems to be a catch-all for febrile infant convulsions.

A final method of disease causation which should be mentioned is contagion, which seems to occur only in the case of epilepsy. Epilepsy may develop if a child has "rabbit" at an early age but is not effectively cured. However, the place where an epileptic falls in a fit becomes contagious and if the path or ground is not burned, others who pass by the same spot may become afflicted.

2.3. DIVINATION

Not all sicknesses require divination to determine the causes of the disorder. As previously noted, severity of symptoms and duration of the complaint seem to distinguish between "natural" and "unnatural" conditions. An unnatural condition is likely to provoke questions regarding causation and thus require divination. When questions of ultimate causation arise, a diviner (*sɔrɔ*) may be consulted (*bikiaru*: consultation, "an asking"). In Pehunko diviners include Muslim *alifa* who use techniques of divination involving the Koran such as *ya sim* where a stick is held between the pages of the Koran; the name of the suspected guilty party is called (four times for a woman, three for a male) and Bariba state that the pages will grab the stick if the correct name is called. Non-Muslim diviners employ a number of techniques of divination. Primary among these are throwing and reading cowry shells; reading dregs of millet beer left in a gourd; and reading sand thrown on the ground.

The most powerful diviners are members of spirit cults, particularly the *sambani* cult (see Chapter 5) who are alleged to be clairvoyant, whether in or out of a trance state. Members of another cult, *bukakaaru*, on the other hand, can sometimes read the future or determine causation of misfortunes while in a trance, which only occurs during cult dances, while the musicians are playing. Only the *sambani* diviners, then, can be approached at any time for a consultation. In those non-Muslim Bariba villages which have a special person, usually a woman, responsible for communing with the ancestors (*bungi*: spirit person, also *bunkɔsɔ*), people seeking a diviner may consult the *bungi* at a house uniquely designated for that purpose and the diviner will request information from the dead. Pehunko did not have a *bungi* and in fact, most of the surrounding villages had no officiating *bungi*, allegedly because it is now hard to find people willing to take responsibility of replacing those *bungibu* who have died.

In all cases, those who consult a diviner must bring a sacrifice, usually fowl; however, a serious divination may require a bull. Diviners are, of course, consulted for other misfortunes than sickness; for example, one Pehunko Bariba consulted for the death of three bulls in a row – the diviner suggested jealousy among neighbors of his involvement with a United Nations draft animal project, and the consulter has since moved to another village. Another consultation involved a child who was particularly cross and irritable and the child's mother sought to determine whether it was his character, and illness, or due to human intervention. Theft is another type of incident which often leads to divination.

Most divinations regarding sickness are private affairs, sometimes involving only the afflicted individual, and more often, involving the immediate family (or such family as is in residence with the sufferer). Suspicious deaths may, however, provoke more extensive participation among kin of the deceased. Divinations are not routinely held when a death occurs – as one diviner explained:

> A person chooses his death before he is born. Therefore if you die a death which is not likely to be the death you chose, your kin will know you died an unnatural death and they will consult a *soro* to find out how you died.

The interpretation of a natural as opposed to an unnatural death permits a certain flexibility in determining the need for a consultation; those deaths most certain to be perceived as natural are deaths of infants and small children and deaths of old people. However, repeated deaths of small children in one family or of one mother may be cause for suspicion either of sorcery or an *abiku* child (cf. Maclean 1976; Gillies 1976 for similar beliefs among Yoruba, Ogori respectively). An *abiku* is a child with mystical powers who dies and is reborn in the body of each succeeding child unless steps are taken to prevent the child from reappearing.

Of those divinations which received widespread attention in Pehunko during the research period, both involved cases of suspected sorcery (see page 27). However I was unable to obtain the results of those divinations due to outright denials by family members of having obtained an answer from the diviner. In each case, village gossip had it that the head of household had so much "evil on his hands" that his enemies were numerous and anyone might have attempted to seek revenge against the head of household through afflicting the victim. In one case the head of the household was the chief Muslim priest for the village; in the other he was the eldest son of the former village chief. No public accusations were proffered in these or any other cases during the term of the project. (I was unable to ascertain whether public accusations were held in the prerevolutionary period; the village chief apparently dealt with such disputes on occasion but I have no empirical data on this topic.)[6]

Public consultations do occur in some instances. One public divination which was held involved a regional epidemic of measles. In this event, a diviner was consulted to explain the occurrence and offered a remedy to reduce the extent of the misfortune. Thus the village of Tobre, 14 kilometers from Pehunko, consulted a diviner who ordered all the children of the village to have their heads shaved in a special design in order to protect them from illness and a skull was placed on a pole outside the village limits to serve as a *kangi*, an object or medicine used for group protection. Another sort of public divination which has not been held since the Revoution of 1972 involves the crying of the fetish rocks of Pehunko. Customarily, a certain Bariba family is responsible for listening to the rocks and interpreting the meaning of their signals to the village. The rocks in the past served as portents for village-wide harvest failures, epidemics and other misfortunes. However, no public interpretations of omens have been offered in the post-revolutionary period due to government restrictions on traditional ceremonies and rituals.

2.4. THE USE OF SUBSTANCES

The role of human intervention in sickness causation and in healing is predicated on the knowledge and techniques of substance manipulation. Skillful use of substances may therefore enhance a person's power, whether the substance is used for good or malevolent purposes (see pages 37 and 38.) Words, or incantations, may then be combined with the substances for heightened effect. Substances range from inanimate objects (rock, earth, metal) to roots, leaves, bark, animal parts, grasses, seeds, and so forth. The principals on which these substances are presumed to work vary. Where substances are intended for harmful purposes, it seems most often that the principle of "contagious magic" applies. That is, whatever the sorcerer "does to a material object will affect equally the person with whom the object was once in contact, whether it formed part of his body or not" (Frazer 1922:11–12). Bariba will advise that at dusk, all personal and household property should be brought into the house or they might be employed in poisons. (Poisons are not necessarily ingested although the Bariba are known for these too, but may be buried, hidden, etc.) For example, the porridge stirring stick, pots, items of clothing, hair, fingernails, earth where a person urinated, can all be used against one. Similarly, if an unseen voice calls and greets a Bariba, he/she should not reply without knowing who is speaking or the respondent's voice may be captured and used to cause the owner harm.

A popular form of sorcery between co-wives is for one to steal the other's menstrual rags and use them in preparing a product to cause some affliction. One such procedure involves washing the rags in the river which never dries up so that her menses will flow continuously. Much of Bariba healing and sorcery operate in general according to the principle expounded initially by Frazer that "things act on each other at a distance through a secret sympathy" (Frazer 1922:12).

A wife may render her husband impotent by wearing a special leather belt with an amulet containing some portion of his body and calling his name, whenever the husband attempts to have sexual relations with one of the other wives. (This example is taken from a case in Kouande where a man divorced his wife and sent her home for this reason.) Additionally, a person's footprint can be captured and used in sorcery and less directly, objects may be buried or hidden with the intent of working on some portion of the victim's body; for instance, a jealous woman was alleged to have buried a poisoned metal spike under a path where her co-wife would walk, causing the co-wife to become afflicted with a grotesquely swollen leg.

Most Bariba are concerned with protective measures or counter-sorcery products, and in many households, the elderly men and women are responsible for fabricating such prophylactics as amulets, which may contain powdered substances, paper with writing from the Koran (in Muslim families); rings or bracelets cooked in a special brew over which incantations have been pronounced; and packets with a base of dried grasses, which are burnt and the smoke protects against sorcerers. Protective devices are also sought against enemies in war, wild animals, snakes, and so forth. Because of the prevalence of discussions on the subject of sorcery, I made repeated attempts to determine the frequency of actual sorcery accusations; however, although on occasion a person was identified to me as a witch or sorcerer, no instances of public accusations came to light. When asked what an individual does if he/she becomes aware that a sorcerer is attacking informants replied that a person in those circumstances will prepare or have prepared a counter-poison or follow the instructions of a diviner but will not necessarily accuse the attacker even if the identify is known. It seems possible to me that the lack of accusations is a recent phenomenon, related to the increasingly stringent government restrictions on customary law and ritual. In contemporary times, accusations may either be rare or so secretive that an outsider would have difficulty obtaining information on the subject. It does seem clear, though that if, because of a dispute or the deathbed words of someone, a sorcerer is known, the reaction depends on the strength of the victim or victim's relatives. If the sorcerer is stronger, the revenge would be left to God; if not, a counter-poison may be prepared.

If a person has been identified as a sorcerer, in the future, others will be wary of the person and protect themselves. For example, a young woman of Doh was alleged to cause harm and had been held responsible for various misfortunes from her childhood. Other women who had grown up with her remembered that as children, they were warned not to walk on the same path with her or play with her. As an adult, she had difficulty finding someone to marry; it seemed that every man with whom she came in contact died. Finally, she married but her husband died within three months. This woman was not formally accused of witchcraft or sorcery but was avoided in the village; one pregnant women who encountered her on the road prepared an anti-sorcery product to wash in immediately upon arriving home, in order to protect herself and her baby.

2.5. MEDICINES

I have already noted that the line between a poison and a medicine may be tenuous. A horse's tail, to cite one example, may be used to bring back the dead; to accelerate a delivery; or cause a sickness, when the sorcerer flicks the tail and calls the victim's name. Nonetheless, for analytical purposes it seems accurate to distinguish a poison, intended to cause harm, from a medicine, defined as "any substance used as part of a response to illness in the expectation that some of its power will augment that of the patient" (Glick 1967:38). Medicines frequently operate via the principle of homeopathy, or imitation; that is, "like produces like." Accordingly, medicines work by producing or representing an imitation of the desired result; in other words, the underlying assumption is that an effect resembles its cause.

Examples of cures deriving from this principle abound. To describe a few, a baby with weak legs may be washed in an infusion of small prickly leaves. The baby will acquire strong limbs and learn to walk quickly because the spines of the leaves will prick endlessly so that the baby will always want to rise up, not to sit down. Similarly, to wean a recalcitrant child, a medicine is prepared from an herb which produces milky sap or from a tree whose bark exudes a milky liquid, both saps resembling breast milk. A preventive medicine for measles or smallpox involves drinking water from a gourd which is covered with bumps like pustules, and a cure for flatulence is to drink an infusion prepared from a leaf which grows in a folded shape; this infusion will cause the anus to remain shut like the leaf. In obstetrical care, a prime example of the homeopathic principle is the procedure of dropping a medicine gourd from the head of the woman so that the baby may "fall" as the gourd fell; sometimes the birth attendant cries "*baraka*," "a blessing," as the gourd hits the ground, to represent the blessing when the baby is actually born. Similarly, a midwife may remove a dirtdauber insect's nest from the wall, crush it and rub it on the parturient's abdomen because "the dirtdauber has no children of its own, yet it removes them from a nest. May the midwife likewise remove the child from the stomach of its mother."

Not all medicines are based on the homeopathic principle. Many involve a complicated mixture of components: to accelerate labor, for instance, the special medicine of one midwife consists of the following ingredients, prepared as indicated:

The Brown Powder: Slowly toast a whole mouse in an earthenware pot over a low fire. (Stir frequently.) When it is very dry, grind the mouse on a grinding stone.

The Black Powder: Slowly toast a whole viper in an earthenware pot over a low fire. Follow instructions for mouse.

Dosage: in case of slow labour, give small quantity of brown powder in some water in a gourd, followed in a few minutes by same quantity of black powder.

The function of most medicines, especially those which work by imitative means, seems to be to compensate for a deficit in the individual and to bolster the ill person against the forces of the disease. Medicines come in a variety of forms. These include:

Tim: Generic term for medicine, also medicine to rub on the body.

Tiwaaru: Medicine to soak; the water is used in a sauce or drunk straight.

Tisu: Medicine to wash with.

Timbuuru: Medicine in powder, such as ground roots, to ingest, usually in sauce or gruel, sometimes snuff.

Duku: Medicine to burn which heals or protects by smoke.

In addition, scarring may be utilized to relieve pain and swelling and certain conditions such as sprains, bruises, "ampoule." Bad abcesses may be treated by cupping using a cow's horn placed over many tiny knife cuts (*ba wi kaho gira*, they planted a horn on him.) After cupping, for 15 minutes or so, the "bad blood" is removed. (See M. Last in Loudon 1976 on related terminology and practice among the Hausa.)

The type of medicine used depends on the disorder; a combination of forms may be employed simultaneously or consecutively in treatment of one condition. In obstetrics, medicines to wash in and to ingest in powder form are particularly preferred but infusions are also prescribed.

Bariba, then, believe sicknesses to be caused by malevolent agents, either human or non-human, who bring their power to provoke affliction to bear against the strength of the victim. Few sicknesses are considered "natural;" usually a disorder is attributed to the illwill of another individual who has tapped the power of substances to cause harm. The victim's response, correspondingly, is to attempt to protect himself and possibly to retaliate by the same means. The victim may treat himself, or herself, or may seek assistance from more knowledgeable persons, depending on personal circumstances; often an elderly male or female relative of the household will be consulted first, followed by respected neighbors, and in the case of a prolonged affliction, specialists of regional fame may be consulted.

What, in summary, does it mean to a Bariba to be "sick?" First, sickness refers to a state of abnormality or deviation; a sick person is not in a state of well-being. A sick individual may be designated as such by a general term (*u barɔ*: he/she is sick) or specifically (*u bwisirubarɔ*: he/she has abcess sickness; *u busuku barɔ*: she has measles). Other sicknesses do not include the generic term *barɔ*, for example *u kesukumɔ*: he has diarrhea, or *u tunra mɔ*: he has a cough. A person may be labelled as sick whether or not he/she is capable of continuing routine daily tasks; however, it is at the point where such responsibilities cannot be accomplished that a sickness receives serious attention, such as consultation with a diviner. Exceptions to this are appearance of striking symptoms such as a feeling of being gripped in the chest and unable to breathe (indicating sorcery) which may provoke an immediate consultation to determine the cause of the complaint and appropriate treatment.

Reviewing the chart of symptoms on page 25, one finds that the major causes invoked to explain sickness include God, spirits, sorcery, witchcraft and breach of taboo. However, it is important to emphasize that not all conditions are immediately deemed due to malevolent intervention nor is causation always explicitly contemplated. Gravity or severity of symptoms and prolonged duration of the disorder are critical in leading to a concern with causation, divination and consultation with specialist practitioners.

Obstetrical complications fit generally into the pattern of beliefs and practices regarding sickness with the exception that intrinsically, pregnancy and delivery are not considered pathological processes. Pregnancy is considered a perilous state, requiring attention to certain taboos and recommended behaviors; however, until an abnormality or complication presents itself, pregnancy and delivery are not categorized as afflictions parallel to such disorders as "*ampoule*," hernia, measles, syphilis, and so forth. If a complication does arise, it is viewed within the general context of sickness causation (that is, caused by powerful pathological agents) and treated with preparations from the array of forms of treatments which comprise Bariba medicine but the pharmacopeia is relatively unique to obstetrical complaints.[7]

Pregnancy, then, is considered a normal state and a reasonable range of complaints of pregnancy are also considered with the normal order of events. Complaints of pregancy do not require divination or discussion of ultimate causation, and are treated by home remedies or possibly by a particularly knowledgeable friend or neighbor if the complaint is not responsive to family efforts. The most common explanation for complications of labor and delivery, from among the typical causes invoked to explain sickness, is witchcraft. Other explanations such as sorcery, breach of taboo, or unconfessed adultery may be invoked on occasion but the most readily suspected cause of an obstetrical complication is witchcraft. This witchcraft is manifest *in utero* in the form of witch babies, who seek to harm or kill their mother. One possible effect of this explanation is that accusations of witchcraft are not common in cases of obstetrical complications because the existence and malevolent actions of a witch baby are believed to derive from God, not from human efforts to cause harm. However, if a woman experienced repeated obstetrical complications (or delivery of witch babies) a diviner might be consulted to determine the reason for God's displeasure.

In the introduction to this chapter, the hypothesis was put forward that decisions regarding the utilization of alternative medical services are largely derived from the diagnosis of the problem at hand and that treatment of a disorder is related to ideas of sickness causation. Correspondingly, in the event of obstetrical complications, the possibility of witchcraft as a causative factor will be expected to influence the actions of parturients, their families and birth attendants in selecting therapeutic options in that the practitioner or service selected for treatment must be considered competent to treat the disorder, as it is diagnosed. Logically then, a specialist in obstetrical complications will be expected to possess an armamentarium designed to confront witchcraft in a delivery setting.

CHAPTER 3

BELIEFS AND PRACTICES SURROUNDING REPRODUCTIVE PROCESSES

The preceding chapter considered the range of beliefs, values and expectations that comprise major assumptions upon which therapeutic choices are based in Bariba society. In this chapter, one particular dimension of Bariba culture will be presented and discussed – that is, values, beliefs and practices regarding reproductive processes. An understanding of these processes, which include menstruation, conception, abortion, menopause, and sterility is pertinent to this study because of the role which ideal constructs regarding reproduction play both in influencing and justifying choices which arise in relation to various reproductive processes and associated events.

In Chapter 1, it was suggested that "people usually *do* have choices to make, not the least the choice whether to conform to the appropriate norm and role expectations ... " (Heath 1976:176). Further, individuals are postulated to make choices derived from wants, goals and values which comprise alternatives provided in the context of a particular culture. In the present chapter, a consideration of cultural definitions of reproductive processes will illustrate the body of "guidelines" which a Bariba woman acquires during childhood, adolescence, and as a young married woman and upon which decisions regarding obstetrical care may be based and categorized as appropriate. Although such decisions may appear to be sudden, or based on an on-going situation, the decision moment is actually the endpoint of a process in which a range of expectations, past experiences, and current events and alternatives are evaluated.

This discussion is primarily based on information acquired from women. Originally it was assumed that it would be productive to interview both men and women regarding the issue under consideration. However, men consistently referred questions to elderly women whom they claimed to be more knowledgeable. This is not to imply that men had no beliefs or values regarding reproduction but that due to problems inherent in this society in a female interviewer persistently questioning men regarding reproduction, most information, if not otherwise specified, is derived from women.

3.1. MENSTRUATION AND CLITORIDECTOMY

Every Bariba girl is expected to undergo a clitoridectomy prior to her first menstruation. Currently, girls are circumcized at about the age of 6 or 7; young women aged 18 to 20 claim to have been circumcized at ages 8 to 10 and older women state that girls used to undergo the operation when they were much "bigger," closer to the onset of menarche. Traditionally, girls wore no clothes, only beads at the waist, until after the clitoridectomy ceremony. Attempts to obtain explanations for the necessity of the clitoridectomy elicited only the remarks that (1) if a woman retains her clitoris, when she delivers a baby, the baby will touch the clitoris and die; and (2) if a woman has a clitoris, other women will mock her "thing." Men and women allege that a woman who has not had the clitoridectomy will never find a husband and will be ashamed all her life. Briefly, the procedure is as follows: (based on examples reported from the villages of Doh and Pehunko)

(1) Each year when the millet flowers bloom (December), little girls are grouped by neighborhood and/or clusters of those "whose parents are ready." There may be as many as ten groups. Each group eats together, going from house to house to taste a dish. There has never been a girls' "camp" outside the village as there was 20 years ago for boys.

(2) On the day of the ceremony, the girls go to warn the patron spirits of the village and pray at their site (e.g., the black rocks of Pehunko.) Subsequently, their heads are shaved as a symbol of purification. At mid-morning, the girls begin to dance in a circle, singing verses which they repeat after one of the supervising adults. One by one, the girls are grabbed from the circle and cut, with one person holding their feet and another the chest; meanwhile, the others keep singing. As each is cut, the adults cry "a blessing, she has come out of shame," a remark also made at the boy's circumcision ceremony. If the girl starts to cry, an adult stuffs a fruit in her mouth (one sort for aristocrats, another for commoners) and the girl is given gruel with medicine to prevent fainting. When all the girls have been cut, they are washed and a dressing of chewed bark and butter, molded into a form to hold the wound in shape and prevent scarring is set in place. The girls are then shown how to wear rags to absorb the bleeding. After about two weeks of having the wound cleaned twice daily, the groups of girls meet again and bury their rags toward the west and run away from the grave without looking back, to ensure that the clitoris does not grow back. They then dress in their best clothes and mothers' jewelry and traipse from house to house receiving greetings and gifts of small sums of money. The circumcizer (*sinburo*) is paid in cash, the amount varying depending on whether the client is a commoner or aristocrat. No group ceremonies were held; girls in Pehunko were operated on individually or in 2's or 3's although small groups did go calling together. Accounts vary as to whether in the past, girls slept together at an old woman's house or merely ate together and were washed together daily.

The girls did not receive sex education at this time; rather, via songs and chants they are urged to behave as dutiful, well-behaved women and to adhere to certain taboos while recovering from the clitoridectomy. Neither are the girls informed regarding menstruation, although the clitoridectomy serves in one respect as a model for behavior when a girl begins to menstruate. At that time, a girl may be astonished to find blood flowing from herself and will ask an aunt, grandmother, or occasionally her mother, for the meaning of this occurrence. She will then be told to wear a rag as she did after the clitoridectomy and to wash the rags in the same way as she did then. (In fact, menstruation is referred to euphemistically as "on the rag.") Some girls were told when shown how to wash the rags for post-clitoridectomy use to remember this time later but with no fuller explanation than that. Many women say in retrospect that they were afraid at their first menstruation but didn't even tell their mothers or aunts, out of embarrassment. They remembered the rags and had observed older sisters or other women occasionally drying rags or overheard conversations regarding menstrual problems, and took care of themselves.

The fact that the girls do not publically announce the onset of menstruation was remarked by one indigenous midwife during a discussion of marriage ages; she noted that it would be impossible to adhere to a rule regarding marriageability in relation to menarche because so often one doesn't know a girl has begun to menstruate for several months. Taboos associated with menstruation are learned subsequently, and include the prohibition against sexual relations, against entering the chief's room, and against cooking or preparing certain foods such as shredded yam (*wassa-wassa*), a food which "likes cleanliness." In addition, women should not do the wash or their menses will cease before they grow old, which is a serious problem. Women are also prohibited in general from touching or preparing medicines, or other substances while menstruating because their contact will destroy the power of the medicine. This prohibition greatly affects the potential for women to acquire both competence and prestige as healers since they must reach menopause before acquiring the freedom to work consistently in this domain. In principle, women could work with medicines between menstrual periods. However, in reality, they may be prohibited from doing so. For example, I went to call on the chief with an European man; during the visit, the chief took out his poisoned arrows to show the man and I reached for one and began to examine it. With an expression of disgust, the chief took it away from me, remarking to one of his elders that I might be menstruating. I said that I was not; no one responded to this inappropriate comment directly but after sending several small boys out of the room, the chief commented that you couldn't believe a woman when she said she was not menstruating and in general it would be better to keep women and powerful substances out of contact with each other.

3.2. CONCEPTION

Producing numerous healthy offspring, "as many as God will send," is a primary goal of both husband and wife in a Bariba family (see Chapter 4), as throughout rural Africa. Although conception is believed to require both the man and the woman, it is the male contribution which intrinsically stimulates the development of the fetus; if a woman produces only girls, however, the fault is hers.

In general, the women attributed a role in conception to God, man, and woman, and one informant added Muslim saints. The underlying assumption was that man and woman come together with the help of God and may or may not produce a child. It is as if God "charges" the substances of man and woman to bring them to life as a fetus. To several informants, a woman contains eggs in her body which the substance of man enters, to produce a child; each egg *must* become a child. That is why contraception cannot work until a woman has had all the children waiting in her eggs; she cannot stop until the process is complete. This belief was recorded both in response to direct questioning and spontaneously when the following incident occurred. A woman about 35 years old with five children was visiting me with her 2-year-old. Two old men came to call; they greeted the woman and in the course of the conversation which followed, asked her where her "baby" was. She pointed out the 2-year-old as her baby. They then urged her to have another now. She remarked that she had five living boys and although she would like a girl, she would rather stop having babies and engage in trade. The men sternly told her that unless she had used up her eggs, she would be obliged to continue having babies.

Conception is not believed to be more likely during any particular time of the month; however, sexual relations are prohibited during menstruation. Another variant explanation of the process of conception refers to sexual relations – after sexual intercourse, the semen of the man remains inside the woman until her menstruation, whereupon the blood and semen flow out together and are expelled. If pregnancy occurs, the blood and semen remain inside the woman and are incorporated into the fetus. This explanation surfaced in discussions regarding menopause, when women stated that a menopausal woman should not have sexual relations because the semen would have no means of being expelled. Thus it would remain in the body and cause her stomach to swell. Tumors of the uterus or stomach region may also be attributed to post-menopausal intercourse. However, although everyone seemed knowledgeable regarding menopausal women and sex, some were not familiar with the idea that the fetus is produced from blood and semen; others, when the blood and semen hypothesis was presented to them, considered it and said it could be correct, but only God knew.

Most women, whatever their belief regarding the original substance of the fetus, claim that the fetus develops within the woman via the food which the mother eats (although one midwife claimed that the fetus would develop regardless of the diet of the mother). The fetus is believed to hang suspended in a sac in a cavity which stretches from sternum to pelvis, so that the food circulates around the fetus and is hence absorbed or eaten. (A baby with a Mongolian spot – a temporary patch of dark pigmentation which may appear in the sacro-lumbar region, especially among dark-skinned peoples – was allegedly burned by overly hot food eaten by the mother.)

The fetus, then, does not develop within a special organ comparable to the uterus, which is permanently anchored within the woman's body. Rather, the fetus hangs suspended in the central cavity of the woman, but covered with a membrane referred to as *marutu*. This term is significant because of preferred means of coping with obstetrical complications and also in the preparation of certain obstetrical medicines, of which more is discussed later. *Marutu*, analyzed etymologically, means: *maru* (to be born); *tu* (that which makes). *Tu* is that which one uses to make, as in *uku tu*, that which one uses to cultivate. In common parlance, *marutu* refers to the place where the child rests within the mother but the term used by specialists seems to refer to the amniotic sac, fragments of which can sometimes be observed during the delivery. Because the fetus and placenta are alleged to rest together inside the *marutu*, both the fetus and placenta should be expelled simultaneously. The expulsion of the *marutu* is not a matter of concern but delay in expulsion of the placenta, as part of the fetus, results in consternation (see Chapter 7). According to several midwives, the most effective Bariba medicine for a retained placenta was made from the *marutu* of a mare. This substance had to be collected in a certain village, Banikoara, when the mares foal, at one time during the year. (It is not clear to me whether they were really using placental fragments.) The technique of preparing this medicine seems to be lost, at least among midwives of the Kouande District. Moreover, knowledge of the more esoteric meaning of *marutu* (sac, as opposed to 'place where child rests') seems limited to certain very old matrones.

3.3. DEVELOPMENT OF FETUS

The stages of development of the fetus are described uniformly by all informants. During the first three months, the girl fetus resembles a frog and the boy a lizard. In four months, all its parts are present, but in miniature and thereafter, the parts increase in size until the pregnancy is at term (10 lunar months.) In the seventh month, the fetus is visible, though small. Special precautions are taken with such a child; for example, the water in which it is washed is saved for two more months and then thrown out. The baby born at eight months, on the other hand, is not called "a delivery" at all, but a miscarriage, and is expected to die. It is not even a baby – it is an abnormal creature, whose body has reverted to blood, with no form. As one woman said, it is as if you basted some sewing and before you sewed it on the machine, you took out the basting threads so that nothing was left but the pieces. This belief is intriguing because it has been recorded for other ethnic groups and regions (for instance, in Cebu and for Appalachian whites). Another notable point raised by the stages of development issue is that women seem to be expected to keep track of the months of their pregnancy, although in personal encounters, women often claimed they did not know. Possibly disclaiming knowledge was due to embarrassment. Midwives state that although a person (including the mother) cannot know the day or week of the anticipated delivery, the midwife who has a pregnant woman in her household and can observe her growth can estimate in which month she is ready to deliver.

3.4. CONTRACEPTION

As far as I was able to determine, the Bariba pharmacopeia does not include a contraceptive to be ingested or inserted. The forms of contraception preferred are for the women to wear a special amulet on a belt around her waist (these are fabricated by men) or most directly, for her to separate herself from her husband; she might, for example, go home to her family during the nursing period of her first children. The former Land Chief of Pehunko proclaimed on this subject: "a woman who doesn't want to have a child might chew *kama* (potash) and spit it on the grave of the ancestors and pray. But she would do better not to go to the room of her husband."

In fact, contraception is rarely sought, given the local emphasis on childbearing, except when a prior child is too young to be weaned, or sometimes in the case of schoolgirls. (Sexual relations while nursing are prohibited due to the explanation that semen will pollute the breastmilk and cause sickness in the nursing child.) Other than through abstinence, then, contraception seems rarely to be attempted. However most women do nurse their babies at least to the age of 20-months and abstain from sexual relations during this period, resulting in an effective child spacing system.

3.5. ABORTION

Abortion, contrastingly, is more frequently encountered, although it is abhorrent to Muslims and non-Muslim Bariba alike on grounds of destroying life and being "unnatural," counter to the ideal role of women, and so forth. There are several sets of circumstances in which abortion might be deemed necessary, or at least, the lesser of two evils. One is that mentioned above – when a woman becomes pregnant before her child is old enought to be weaned (20 months approximately). Should she not have an abortion, others will know that her husband came to her room and she will be ashamed. A Pehunko woman who became pregnant when her previous child was 16 or 17 months old was much discussed, if not mocked. Another situation where abortion might be attempted is that where a woman becomes pregnant while her husband is away from home, or when a woman becomes pregnant and cannot name the father. The latter instance is one of the most shameful occurrences conceivable to Bariba because a child must know its father's name and clan to receive its own name. A baby with an unknown father would receive mocking greetings from others such as "hello baby . . . baby who?"

In contemporary times, abortions are perhaps most common among schoolgirls, who seem to get caught in conflicting goals – to finish exams, to have a child, to comply with a schoolmaster's importuning. One death occured in Kouande in 1976–77 from an abortion attempted by a secondary schoolgirl, while seven deaths were publically known in the provincial capital of Natitingou. In the customary approach, abortions were provoked by ingesting such products as an infusion of barks or leaves or indigo dye mixes. Usually a woman who wanted an abortion would secretively consult an elderly woman of her own family (or possibly her husband's family, if he knew) and request a medicine.

No medicines to insert in the vagina were used. Currently, in addition to the customary medicines, women use kerosene, gasoline, and European medicines, particularly quinine products. Most deaths have occurred from overdoses of quinine. This information was obtained from schoolgirl informants in Natitingou but further information on products used as abortifacients in rural areas could not be obtained due to the secrecy surrounding this subject. Moreover, the young women who periodically consulted their aged relatives for me regarding such matters might have been misconstrued had they persisted in questioning their relatives regarding means of provoking abortions.

3.6. STERILITY

Conception is said to derive primarily from the man, although the function of the woman's contribution is delineated. Constrastingly, sterility is tacitly assumed to be the fault of the woman, except under certain circumstances. If, for instance, a man has had several wives and none have produced children but at least one has married elsewhere and had children, by deduction, the man is believed to be sterile and should seek treatment. Usually, unless a man is impotent, he is assumed to be capable of fathering children. (Frankenberg and Leeson 1976, describe similar beliefs in Lusaka). If a couple has been married for a year and the woman has not become pregnant, she will probably seek a medicine from a relative or neighbor.

One such case was that of Zalia, who was married at 19, had no children after one year of marriage, and her husband was speaking of taking a second wife. She had a neighbor who treated her "just like a younger sister." This neighbor prepared her a medicine in liquid form, gave it to her in a beer bottle and told her to take it throughout the month, a swig at a time. She became pregnant the second month. If she had not become pregnant, she probably would have consulted a specialist.

Most sterility specialists are old men (few midwives handle sterility cases; see Chapter 5) although one old matrone near Pehunko was noted for her successful treatment of sterile women. This old woman was a leader of a spirit possession cult and was singled out by her penchant for living all alone in a house about one kilometer in the bush from a small village called Fwabwereku. This woman, who looked to be about age 80 at least, was a clairvoyant who threw cowrie shells to read the cause of the sterility. After divining, she would prescribe roots or medicine to wash in to remove the sterility and if conception occurred, the client would then pay her. (This diviner is an example of one who combined divining and herbalist functions.)

Divining in a case of sterility would be expected to elicit a limited number of causes. One cause is simply "mismatched blood" between the man and woman, which prevents conception. A much dreaded cause is the curse of either spouse's father's sister, which is extremely difficult to remove; sorcery can also be responsible for sterility but is less critical because it can be counter-acted, whereas father's sister's curse must be analyzed, retribution offered for the offense, retribution accepted, and so forth. Impotence in a man and more rarely sterility in a woman may be blamed on the mother who let breastmilk drip on the genitals of the nursing child. For this reason, babies should be clothed or covered while nursing. Other explanations for sterility included the belief that a young woman who tried to work as a midwife in a clinic and who had had not children herself would become infertile. The young woman did not conceive after 2½ years and eventualy went to a specialist in another town; she now has a child.

The curse of sterility is perhaps the most dreaded fate to either a man or a woman, as manifest in the burial procedure for a person who dies without children – the lower back of such a person is broken (or beaten) before burial and the person is buried facing west, so that the misfortune may go down with the sun. This grim burial also symbolizes the obscurity and uncertainty brought when the sun sinks in the west, with the west generally representing unhappiness and misfortune.

The review of beliefs and practices regarding reproductive processes presented thus far underscores the importance attributed to fertility and the concomitant affirmation of conception and birth as events of primary value. Correspondingly, deliberate abortion and sterility – both of which represent a symbolic opposition to fertility and birth are defined as abhorrent, although socially acceptable explanations for their occurrence exist and can be drawn upon, depending on the situation. Thus abortion may be a necessary option to preserve honor although in a larger sense it is a shameful choice. In contrast, sterility is not a deliberate choice like abortion, but it can be explained in terms of the culpability of the individual (breach of taboo) or fate (mismatched blood, God). The concept of sterility as a curse highlights the opposing concept of conception and birth as blessings. It is noteworthy that the Bariba language includes three words for vagina, specifically (1) the pre-circumcized vagina (*sinkiru*); (2) the menstruating vagina (*bẽru*), which is also the post-circumcized vagina; and (3) the post-delivery vagina (*koru*), thus illustrating the significance attached to this passageway. The roles of the specialists who deal with these processes are correspondingly valued. In particular, the sterility specialist and the midwife, both of whom make it possible to produce life, are greatly esteemed and it is in regard to this role that they can be perceived as transcending ordinary status categories.

The next chapter, then, will examine the role of women in Bariba society and in particular, women's domain of decision-making responsibility, in order to arrive at an understanding of the role of the matrone as a specialist dealing with reproduction. The chapter will also provide a perspective on the locus of decision-making responsibility which is necessary to a full discussion of factors such as beliefs regarding causation of misfortunes and reproduction which may influence selection of birth assistance.

CHAPTER 4

STATUS AMONG THE BARIBA: THE ROLES AND RESPONSIBILITIES OF WOMEN

Throughout this discussion, the status of Bariba women is assumed to be of critical significance to an examination of birth practices because reproduction is a domain of particular concern to women.[8] "Women's goals are . . . defined by their position in the society as a whole," (Lamphere 1974:100) as are the means which they select to achieve those goals. Correspondingly, the goals of Bariba women regarding reproduction might be expected to derive from their status in Bariba society.

A useful perspective for considering the status of women in Bariba society is that suggested by Rosaldo (1974). Rosaldo states that

> . . . characteristic aspects of male and female roles in social, cultural and economic systems can all be related to a universal, structural opposition between domestic and public domains of activity . . . (Rosaldo 1974:35).

Sanday, writing about this opposition, clarifies that "the domestic domain refers here to those activities performed within the realm of the localized family unit whereas the public domain includes political and economic activities that take place or have impact beyond the localized family unit . . . (Rosaldo 1975:190).

According to Rosaldo, women's status is lowest in those societies where there is a firm differentiation between the domestic and public spheres of activity and where women are isolated from one another, and placed under a single man's authority, in the home. Correspondingly,

> Their position is raised when they can challenge those claims to authority, either by taking on men's roles or by establishing social ties, by creating a sense of rank, order, and value in a world in which women prevail. One possibility for women, then, is to enter the men's world or to create a public world of their own (Rosaldo, 1974:36).

Moreover, Rosaldo suggests that in societies with a clear differentiation between the domestic and public domains, extra-domestic ties with other women are an important source of power and value for women (39). She also notes that the domestic/public opposition supports a general identification of women with domestic life and of men with public life (23–4). Comparably, Paulme in reviewing the status of women in tropical Africa states that overall, the participation of women in the public domain is much less than that of men (Paulme 1960: 7).

Similarly, in the Bariba case it is hypothesized that the degree to which a distinction is manifest between the domestic and public domains is indicative of the status of women in Bariba society, and that "women gain power and a sense of value when they are able to transcend domestic limits" (Rosaldo 1974:41).

Thus the status of Bariba women will be enhanced by extra-domestic ties and activities which enable women to transcend the domestic domain.

4.1. STATUS IN BARIBA SOCIETY

Before focusing on the status of women in Bariba society, stratification in general will be considered briefly. Among the Bariba, status was linked to occupation (Lombard 1965:146), with war, hunting and artisanry representing the major possibilities for increasing one's reknown. Above all these socially differentiated positions came the distinction of aristocrat (*wasangari*) as distinguished from commoner (*baatonu*). Even the label "hunter" does not supercede that of origin of birth, although all Bariba males aspire to be successful hunters, and the true hunters who possess poisons are commoners, of the clan "*tauso*." The second most important line of differentiation, according to Lombard, was that of families serving official function, such as land chiefs allied to nobles, in contrast to those with no customary hereditary political functions.

Among artisans, the blacksmith was accorded highest status (Lombard 1965: 149); this derived from "sa puissance spirituelle qui l'autorisait à manier l'élément naturel le plus dangereux, le feu, et à fabriquer tous les instruments qui avaient pouvoir de vie – les outils agricoles – comme de mort – les armes" (p. 149).[9] According to Lombard, following the blacksmith in prestige were barbers and butchers; barbers, besides coiffing men and sometimes women, also hold responsibility for treating certain illnesses, scarring, head-shaving for ceremonial purposes, and so forth. Lombard (1957) describes the differentiation of artisans as follows:

Artisans	Other Services
blacksmiths	butchers
barbers	hunters
dyers	praise-singers
leatherworkers	gravediggers
gourd engravers	
weavers	
wicker workers	
wood sculptors	
potters	

According to Lombard, status is differentiated by the Bariba on the basis of sex, age, profession, birth, education, marital alliance and political function. Remarking on the complex indices for status differentiation, he states that "chaque attitude de la vie quotidienne tendait toujours à préciser un statut et il n'y avait pas de contract entre individus qui ne fut au préalable pour l'un la reconnaissance de son infériorité hiérarchique, sinon de sa dépendence" (177).[10] It is especially significant, then, that in this hierarchy of statuses, he lists no women's occupations except "potter." Of pottery, he notes that throughout

West Africa, pottery is a female trade, perhaps due to a symbolic link between women, earth and fertility. Like blacksmiths, potters have rites, prohibited behavior, and special customs. The trade is strictly transmitted by a mother to daughter apprenticeship; potters also may serve a healing role, specializing in finding and preparing clays for treatment of diarrheas and for those (especially women and children) who crave clay.

Perhaps because his attention was focused on formal political positions, Lombard did not fully investigate the statuses filled by women, although he touched briefly on this issue. Fundamentally, however, he was correct in stating that sex is a basic determinant of status in that a woman could never aspire to an elevated social position. Her position evolves primarily within the family, according to her age, order of birth and, as a married woman, ranking among wives; a married woman's status reflects that of her husband. A woman's status in general, then, is ascribed rather than achieved. There exist, however, rare exceptions where personal initiative may modify a woman's social position. A woman who acquires sufficient wealth and demonstrates authority and organizational ability might become head of a woman's group such as the associations which provide food and entertainment for high-ranking strangers.

Among noble Bariba, the chief's oldest sister holds the sole titled position; no parallel positions exist among commoners.[11] This woman, known as the Yɔ̃ Kogi, occupied the one political function allocated to aristocratic women. Her responsibilities included giving the order for the shaving of the heads of young aristocratic children who were about to receive a noble name; Yɔ̃ Kogi also chose the name for each child. It is said that on the naming day, the chief's sister is like the chief so that one must remove one's shoes before entering her courtyard as if showing respect to a chief.

A commoner woman may hold the title of *gooyankuko*, the inherited position as the leader of funeral chants who must initiate the ceremony which precedes the beating of the drums at a death. Among Muslim Bariba, three titled hereditary positions exist: these include Ya and her two helpers Taba-Taba and Yɔ̃ Kuura. These three elderly women must be present at all Muslim baptisms and weddings, where their functions consist of washing the bride and groom, verifying the virginity of the bride and lodging the bride the night before her wedding; Yɔ̃ Kuura also trills the name of the bride and groom as accompaniment to the proceedings. At baptisms, the three attend but only Yɔ̃ Kuura actively participates. Her role is to trill and sing out the name of the child after the Imam prays aloud, citing the new name. Inheritance of these positions varies – Yɔ̃ Kuura of Pehunko claims that her mother, her mother's mother, and her mother's grandmother held the position whereas Taba-Taba of Pehunko inherited her position in the classical pattern, from her father's sister. When she dies, the position will be held in turn by her sisters in order of age, and then by their nieces. In interviews with the Muslim title-holders, these women claim that they, together with the chief's sister, were the "important" and respected women of the past "before the revolution." They cited the leaders of women's associations and important female traders as other women held in respect. Both women and men claim that no women were ever consulted politically.

Professional activities also carry the potential for increasing a woman's prestige and affording her a unique identify. Such activities include pottery, already mentioned, and performing female circumcision. Other activities which proclaim a woman's worth are midwifery; spirit cult membership, particularly leadership of a cult; the practice of *bunkɔsɔ*, contacting the dead and transmitting information; and *sɔrɔ*, divining (diviners are usually spirit possession cult members also). (See Chapter 5 for more lengthy discussion of these specializations.) In this regard, Lombard writes "les potières, les matrones, les initiées, et surtout les prêtesses des cultes avaient une influence qui dépassait bien souvent les limites du village ou même de la région, et certaines réputations pouvaient se propager dans tout le pays bariba par l'intermédiare des griots" (143).[12]

All women interviewed agreed that women in the pre-colonial period (and probably this situation persisted in rural areas until the revolutionary period, post-1972) lacked political power and clearly, in contrast to the numerous titled political positions of traditional society, the authority of women could not compare with that of men (cf. Paulme who notes that in tropical Africa, the facts show that it is very rare to find political power vested in a woman [Paulme 1960: 5]).

4.2. POSITION OF WOMEN

The preceding review of stratification in Bariba society suggests that a clear demarcation exists between the "domestic" and the "public" domains and that the affairs of women are largely restricted to the domestic sphere, with the exception of midwives, spirit cult members and spirit communicators, and to a lesser extent potters, whose activities do transcend the household domain. The differentiation between the domestic and public domains will become even more evident after a closer examination of women's roles; correspondingly, the significance of those statuses which do permit women to participate in the public domain will be underscored. The areas to be considered in this discussion include women's roles in subsistence, in politics, in the domestic unit and in health care. This information is primarily based on participation-observation and unstructured interviewing undertaken in the villages of Pehunko and Kouande.

4.3. ECONOMIC SUBSISTENCE

In 1976–77, the national government of Benin adopted a new constitution which included a provision stating that women are equal to men. Discussion of this provision in the various village councils in the north elicited some dubious comments by men, who remarked that possibly female civil servants could be said to be equal to male civil servants, but the Bariba *women* did not work, thus in what sense could they be considered equal? Other men did not issue such a harsh review. Most concluded that women were not equal but that they did perform important functions, foremost among these being childbearing and child-raising. Women also play an appreciable role in agriculture, although men seem to show disdain towards the input of women. Not all women participate in the agricultural responsibilities of the domestic unit; if there are several women in a household, at least one will stay home to do domestic tasks and some wives of aristocrats or women from town who married a villager do not go to the fields. Those who work in the fields engage in the following tasks:

1. Bringing seed yams to the fields; only men make mounds and harvest the yams.
2. Seed millet, cut millet heads after the men bend down the stalks, thresh and pound millet.
3. Seed and thresh rice.
4. Seed and harvest corn.
5. Seed and harvest beans.
6. Seed and harvest peanuts.
7. Seed and harvest cotton.
8. Undertake responsibility for all condiment crops (leaves, gumbo, peppers.)
9. Collect karite (shea butter) nuts and make butter.

Women and men seed and harvest millet, rice, corn, peanuts and cotton crops together; women do not weed any crops. The male head of household, sometimes in conjunction with his brothers or sons, makes all decisions regarding time of operations, dealing with contingencies such as bush fires, scavengers, conflicts with neighboring field-workers. Thus although women participate in the majority of agricultural operations, they do not usually have decision-making responsibilities regarding cultivation. This fact is significant in that women lack the access to power which they might acquire from holding authority in the area of subsistence.[13] Rosaldo, for instance, suggests that by control of foodstuffs and economic contributions, women may influence men but Bariba women lack such control and associated influence.

Women do, however, have one special crop for which they are responsible, in addition to sauce and condiment production. Shea butter nuts are the particular province of women; during May and June most women spend all their spare time collecting the nuts, which are parboiled and stored for the rest of the year, to be made as needed into the butter which is a sauce base. Shea butter nuts are especially significant to women, not only as a staple in the diet but because women sell butter in the market, and the profits are uniquely theirs.

Profits from the harveting of cash crops such as peanuts and cotton are held to belong to the head of household and/or male responsible for a particular field, where the family is engaged in a large operation. A husband then should pay taxes, provide food (both market-bought and in the sense that harvested grain, etc. is "provided" by him) and maintain adequate housing for his wives and children and other dependents; in contemporary times, he may pay school fees and clothing for his children or the mother of a child may have responsibilities for clothing. Women are responsible for financing their own clothing, (except for occasional gifts, e.g., at the New Year from a benevolent husband), jewelry, some household necessities such as soap, bought medicines, luxuries for children, and anything which could be classified as a personal item or investment.

Other than by selling butter, women acquire cash by numerous means. Almost all women are petty traders. Female traders elsewhere in West Africa have received attention in anthropological and other literature, in part because of the notable wealth and power of the women involved. Leis, for example, remarked that associations of women in West Africa (and associations of market women, such as those found among Yoruba women, are prominent types of associations) give women considerable power " . . . and they can, to varying extents, even manipulate men or at least stand as virtual equals with them" (Leis 1974:223). Van Allen notes more specifically that:

> A few women can acquire wealth and considerable prestige through trade; women traders in Ghana and Nigeria have amassed capital holdings of £2000 or more. For most women, however, profits are small, providing at best maintenance of their economic position (Van Allen 1976:40).

Very few Bariba women in rural areas manage to amass much capital (Bariba women in towns such as Parakou, capital of the Borgou Province, are more likely to engage in trade on a much larger scale.) However, almost invariably, women sell some product in attempts to acquire a profit, whether the enterprise in restricted to sales on market days or on a daily basis.

An interesting finding in the survey on Bariba women of reproductive age was that all women (119) responded to the question "what work do you do" by describing what they sold, either at home or at the market. Trading activities range from selling prepared food, or a variety of small items (sugar, razor blades, soap, candy) to more indigenous products such as mustard, sponges, cotton thread or homemade soap. (Spinning cotton is a female activity, now progressively limited to older women; men weave the cotton and sell cloth.) Many women who have obtained some mission education crochet or knit baby clothes by commission or to be sold at the market. Plaiting hair is also a means of earning a small sum. Profits from all these activities belong entirely to the woman, who may spend her earnings entirely on household necessities or, if she can save sufficiently, she will probably invest in a larger enterprise, for example, selling pots and pans, bread, or a large array of medicines, beads or other small items. Women may initiate an escalation in vending enterprise by means of a "*tontine*," a sort of revolving credit association wherein a group of 10 or 20 women contribute a regular weekly sum to a communal pot and once a month, or every time a certain sum is reached, a different women takes the total for her own purposes. Men also utilize the *tontine* approach.

Given the fact that elsewhere, as noted above for the Yoruba, associations of female traders have provided women with considerable power, it is worth noting that no such associations exist among the Bariba women. One association, the *yigberu*, does exist, in which women (primarily married women of reproductive age) participate; however, the function of the *yigberu* is primarily to collect wood, prepare food and provide entertainment for village-wide festivities, particularly when dignitaries are visiting and must be appropriately hosted. The head of the *yigberu* (*yaayikpe*) tends to be a woman capable of making decisions, organizing and with income of her own to use for commissions to assistants, for lodging people at her house, and so forth. She as an individual may have significant influence on village women (see, for example, the Case of Sako, Chapter 7) may counsel them, set fashions, act as a role model (for instance, the *yaayikpe* of Pehunko was the only woman to enroll in a Bariba literacy course offered by the national government). However, participation in the *yigberu* does not provide women with political power, an opportunity to increase monetary profits or to act as an interest group.[14]

Petty trade usually does not differentiate status of women or enable a woman to increase her decision-making input in any domain. Once a woman escalates to a large trade, however, her position may be different. Other than the few female traditional functionaries (for example, circumciser, marriage/baptism officials) the most vociferous and respected women in Pehunko included three traders with large investments, one of whom also sold bread. One such woman was a Muslim, whose wealth eventually enabled her to make two trips to Mecca; another held the position of president of women (*yaayigkpe*) whose responsibilities include calling together and supervising all young married women to host visitors, prepare food, clean village buildings, march in demonstrations, etc. Unlike most women, both of these women are outspoken and confident in public gatherings. Other women say of wealthy female traders that they don't "need" men; for this reason men say that a woman who sells a few items to supplement the household income is a good woman but a woman who acquires a large capital to invest will go her own way.

Similarly, woman may inherit from both parents; her mother or her aunt's personal property may come to her but if her father leaves cattle, they will be for a son, even if a daughter is older, unless the dying person specifically declares that the son should give certain cattle to a daughter who had done well. In such a case, men say, a good girl will give her inheritance to a brother to take care of them for her. (one man explained, for example, that his mother bequeathed her cattle to her brother, who later left them to him and his brothers.) On the other hand, a female trader with cattle might buy cattle or keep inherited cattle under her own control by giving them to a Fulbe to herd but not to a close relative.

4.4. POLITICAL ARENA

I have already stated that amidst the plethora of formal titled political positions which comprised Bariba society, none were allocated to women except the position of Yɔ̃ Kogi, the chief's sister, who was responsible for naming aristocratic children. Women, then, did not customarily share in political authority. Regarding the power of women as manifest in influencing political decisions, this is now difficult to evaluate given the current emphasis of the national government on dismantling the traditional political systems. Elderly women claim that no women offer opinions to men, nor are they asked for their opinion. The only exception cited was *bungibu*, those women who communicate with spirits. Via these links with the spirit world, they are owed and receive respect. One might infer that such a woman who wanted to comment on some aspect of warfare, secession, or succession disputes which are alleged to be the realm of men, might do so with impunity but I have no data to confirm this speculation. In the contemporary context (post-1972), each village agglomeration is required to appoint representatives or counselors including a certain number of representatives of women, such as the president of the women of Pehunko. Thus far, most women have been very reluctant to participate in meetings or demonstrations organized by the national government and decisions regarding commune affairs are still spearheaded by men.

4.5. DOMESTIC RELATIONS

4.5.1. *Marriage*

Although the situation appears to be changing, it is still the case that most marriages of rural Bariba girls are arranged, some against the wishes of the girl, and sometimes when she is as young as nine years old. (In one recent case near Pehunko, the grandmother of a nine-year-old promised her to a 20-year-old man.) Girls promised to a chief are sent to live in his household as early as nine or ten but other fiancées don't go to their husband's household until some months after the onset of menstruation (mean 14.3 months; median 7–12 months). According to a sample of 232 women seen at the Cotonou maternity who knew their age, the average age at menarche was 15 (Alihonou, personal communication).

The Bariba are a patrilineal society with virilocality as the characteristic residence pattern. Marriage seems to be relatively unstable (Lombard 1965: 164–6); a woman is alleged always to belong to her family of origin and never to her husband's family, where she is always a stranger. Both a woman and a man have the right to one formal marriage (*kurɔkpaaru*); thereafter, a woman may leave a man and establish residence with another but if the first dies twenty years later, she must sit formal mourning for him. Children always belong to their father and often go to live with him or his brother after the age of six or so, in the case of a separation. Most women say that a woman can leave her husband freely as long as she has produced one or two children; if not, they will say "you've given nothing" and attempt to obtain a judicial settlement.

Bariba men claim a goal of polygamy, with the intent of assuring security in old age, numerous offspring, and increasing prestige, one means of indicating wealth being the number of wives a man can support. In the survey of 119 women of Pehunko, 64% were living in polygamous households; of these 26% were one of two wives; 16% one of three wives, 12% one of four wives, 8% one of more than four wives; and 3% were single or widowed. Women indicated that the number of wives in residence varied according to reproductive status, conflicts, and so forth. Thus if the sample is indicative, a majority of Bariba women are either married into households where they will be a subordinate wife, or will at some point in their marriage, be a co-wife. The rank of a woman in the hierarchy of wives will be shown below to be significant in affecting her workload, freedom of action, income and decision-making authority.

Because no formal mechanisms exist for providing sex education such as have been noted elsewhere in Africa (cf. Turner 1978), girls are introduced to sex by their husbands (or fiancés, although people say that one generation ago girls would not engage in premarital sex). The attitude among women towards sex appears generally to be one of embarrassment (as manifest by giggling and elbowing others during discussions) and the expressed conviction that women do not need sex but men do. Women uniformly stated that brides are reluctant to go to their husband's room and are only interested in sex for procreative purposes, but that a woman *must* accept her husband's advances except if she is menstruating or nursing. (The effect of refusals probably varies according to whether a woman has already borne several children, whether she has co-wives, and so forth.) Further, men state that women are free to approach men for sex as they like, but on the other hand, women reply "who would want to?" Women add, however, that adolescent girls nowadays appear to be more interested in sex than their elders as indicated by how often they become pregnant while unmarried.

4.6. HOUSEHOLD RESPONSIBILITIES

(See Appendix A for demographic data.) The night before her marriage ceremony, a woman is advised by taba-taba, one of the marriage officials, concerning her duties as a wife. She is cautioned to rise early, sweep the courtyard, fill the water jars, get wood for the fires, speak when spoken to, not to wait for the mother-in-law to do something but to do it first, to pray, etc. In a polygamous household, there is a loose division of labor, with the first wife having the responsibility for making the sauce, the second the porridge, and menial tasks delegated to those lowest in the hierarchy. The first wife allocates tasks, oversees daily workload completion, arbitrates problems which arise among women and children. If, in the ideal situation, she has a much lighter workload than the other women, she may well have more time to devote to trade, thus enhancing the means at her disposal to maintain her prestige. Co-wives, according to the statement of ideal behavior, should get along like sisters. In reality, however, much rivalry and jealousy exists. In the case where a man has three wives, for example, it is often said that the first two will join forces to harass the third, giving her all the time-consuming and difficult work to do. Co-wives acquire prestige from their husband's capability to support several wives, as well as from his general status in the community. (The reverse does not appear to be true although a rude, lazy or "shameless" wife is a discredit to her husband. It seems that she is more of a discredit, though, to her own kin.)

In the areas of food preparation and child care, women not only take the initiative but are held to be primarily responsible. Thus bathing, dressing, feeding and medicating children with the end goal of maintaining them in good health is a major role almost exclusively for women. In most circumstances, a woman must ask her husband's permission for other than routine undertakings – thus she should receive permission to make major purchases, voyage, go visiting after dark, attend ceremonies. Where young children are concerned, however, her range of initiative is greater, although a young woman may ask advice of an older co-wife, sister, aunt or friend. Women will, for instance, evaluate the health of a child and decide to take the child to an elderly midwife who specializes in a certain type of treatment (perhaps for fattening or eye infections) without consulting her husband. (The husband may also instigate such treatments if he wishes to intervene.) So, in sum, the major responsibility for keeping a child alive is that of the mother. Some women still ask permission before taking a child to a dispensary but increasingly, it seems that treating a child for common disorders such as fever, intestinal problems or measles at the dispensary is an option which women can draw upon as independently as utilizing an indigenous healer. Where major illness strikes a family, however, particularly when older children or adults are involved, it is the male head of the household who decides what course of action is necessary and who may himself prepare a treatment.

The women with a wealthy and benevolent husband may have slightly more freedom than other women in terms of household responsibilities. Thus a woman with cash input from her husband may take grain to the mill to be ground (most women now do so but some might need to pay from their own savings); buy wood rather than gather it; be able to bring young nieces to live in the household to help with domestic tasks, and so forth. It is interesting to note that currently, as cash crops increasingly provide income for households, even men who give their wives generous sums of money are loathe to pay for firewood, even though it is now ubiquitously for sale. Men argue that because gathering wood is a woman's responsibility, if she wants to buy it instead, she must do so from her own earnings. The position of a wife vis-à-vis her husband is well described in the notebooks of Father Cardot, a French priest who worked for many years among the Bariba. He remarked that:

> The wife does not call her husband by his name, but she gives him a name by which she calls him (e.g., father, master, teacher.) She does not intervene when he is speaking with others, she only speaks if he asks her. The woman is not free in her actions when the husband is there; when he is working, she can go where she wants, but he will ask her every-

thing later. The proverb states: a woman never becomes an adult (*tonduro bukara mɔpai!*) All disputes begin with women; husbands don't like their wives to visit old ladies because the elderly give them bad advice.

The rights of the women depend on the character of the husband; some men never beat their wives. [If he does] if she hasn't done anything serious (such as neglect the children) her parents can take her back.

The wife, then has a certain recourse in leaving her husband. She may also leave for up to a couple of years after the birth of her first two children. The disturbance which this causes him, of course, depends on whether he is polygamous, has a sister living with him, etc. Wives seem more prone to leave a husband due to conflicts with co-wives; for example, in the case of a first wife who left because the second, much younger wife and husband were always together chatting and neglected her over a period of several years. Very rarely, a woman serves in fact as head of her own household. Such women are usually elderly, members of spirit cults or are spirit communicators and are both feared and respected as such, by men and women alike.

A consideration of the role of women would be incomplete without a discussion of the concept of "shame" or *sekuru*. The behavior of women is circumscribed by the code of appropriate behavior and bounded by that which would cause shame and that which would denote propriety. The behavior of both men and women is influenced by notions of propriety but women seem to be particularly tightly regulated in this sense. As Father Cardot noted, women are prohibited from saying the name of their husband (they would 'eat shame' if they did); they also should not say the names of their children or at least the elder two. By doing so they would be demonstrating undue pride, which would show them to be shameless. Women should not discuss reproduction, their husbands, or give their own opinions in a public situation. A woman would also be shamed if she neglected obligations such as gift-giving or attending baptisms or funerals, but these breaches also apply to men. Generally, explanations for why a woman would or would not behave in a certain way are couched in terms of her fear of being perceived as "shameless," and/or lacking in respect, whether respect towards men (older and younger) or women (older or superior in status).

The implication that the status of women is low and that women are in many senses subordinate beings in Bariba society is manifest in proverbs (such as "a woman never grows up"); in the fact that a leaf is named "a woman is not a person;" in notions of expected behavior; and in analyses of observed situations. Women perform necessary functions in agriculture but do not hold decision-making positions; they are almost totally devoid of formal political power; their prestige in the household is greatly derived from that of the husband, and ideally at least, their verbal and behavioral initiative in the household is restricted when the husband is present. One can comprehend, then, the fact that Lombard's 600 page work on the Bariba barely mentions women. However, in the domestic sphere, women have decision-making authority with regard to child care responsibilities and to some extent in food preparation. They also usually retain close ties with their own matrilineal and patrilineal kin (if the husband dies the widow often returns to her brother's household) and these ties can provide leverage in conflicts with the husband. There is no formal divorce, but a woman can choose to leave her husband and expect support from her family if she can show reasonable cause.

In subsequent sections, it will become clear that in contrast to their limited range of authority in more "public" domains, women have the dominant responsibility and decision-making powers in the domain of reproduction, whether regarding clitoridectomy, conception, or labor and delivery. These areas may not be the unique province of women – for example, certain male healers specialize in treating extreme complications of labor, usually where great "power" is deemed necessary, and some sterility specialists are male. Nonetheless, the reproductive processes are primarily under the control of women and it is within this domain that a woman is most likely to succeed in enhancing her position.

The significance of reproduction to Bariba women is closely related to female status in that to every woman, a first pregnancy is indicative of a critical change from the position of young girl to that of mother and an adult woman's reputation and claim to respect is greatly derived from her role as mother of many living children, in particular, sons. Thus a young woman who had been married for three years and never conceived explained her willingness to submit to a pelvic examination by a visiting obstetrician to investigate possible sterility by saying that a woman who has no child would run naked down the street and feel no shame if such an act would cause her to conceive.

One primary means for a woman to enhance her status is to produce numerous healthy children. Behaving as the "ideal wife," amassing capital through trade, laboring industriously in agricultural operations all accrue to a woman's prestige. Healing, the practice of midwifery, membership in a spirit cult, and divining also could enhance a woman's position. As Lombard noted, "il est évident que toute spécialisation professionelle surtout celle touchant à la fécondité et à la naissance, était un supplement de prestige et affermissait le statut particulier de la femme"[15] (Lombard, personal communication). These specialized avenues to prestige will be discussed further in Chapter 5. However, a necessary route to achieving any position of respect and influence for every woman is to be "a mother of children;" and professional specialization does not exempt a woman from the obligation to produce offspring in order to obtain full and meaningful status as an adult woman.[16] Thus a primary goal of most women is to become pregnant and safely deliver healthy children. This goal, though shared by men and women, is to a large extent implemented by women, through the communications of both women of reproductive age and their elders who provide one another with advice and counsel, and diagnosis and treatment regarding the reproductive processes. Midwives, in particular, have a special competence in this area as will be discussed subsequently. To a certain extent, reproduction might be considered part of the domestic domain, in that it is of fundamental significance to the household unit and may be supervised totally from within that unit. However, women, as constituents of a category, share control of reproductive processes and other then in exceptional circumstances, men are excluded from this arena. Thus it seems justifiable to conclude that because they hold responsibility for decisions regarding reproduction – whether as individuals, as members of lay referral systems or as professional specialists – and because while fulfilling those responsibilities they may develop extra-domestic ties, women may in fact transcend the domestic domain.

CHAPTER 5

SOCIOLOGICAL AND CAREER ATTRIBUTES OF MIDWIVES

5.1. HEALERS: MIDWIVES AND MEDICINE PEOPLE

Although all women are expected to have a general competence with reproductive disorders, pregnancy and delivery, certain women specialize in treatment problems associated with such conditions. Via this route, women may acquire renown and respect which are usually the province of men. In order to understand the significance of midwifery as a female professional specialization, it is necessary to consider first the implications of being a healer in Bariba society and then, specifically, the categorization, position, and functions of the midwife.

5.1.1. *Tingi: The Medicine Person*

The Bariba number a large selection of medical practitioners, known in generic terms as "medicine people" (*tingibu*). This term distinguishes them from poisoners, who also use substances but to do evil. Although healers are differentiated from poisoners, healing (and hence the healer) is considered with ambivalence, because of the potential for misuse of power which is involved. Thus in answer to the question "what is a *tingi*?" one informant replied, "it is hard to say because those who have medicine to kill and to heal are both *tingibu*." Correspondingly, one might say "*u tim mowa*!" "Be careful," he has medicine (i.e., is dangerous) but also "*u barɔ, koo wi tim kɛ̃*;" "he's sick, we will give him medicine." The power resides both in the substance and in the person manipulating the substance so that most plants have helpful and harmful properties and uses, depending on the mode of utilization. Because medicines can be used for good or evil, a wise individual will never consult a healer, even one known for competence, unless the healer is a relative and hence trustworthy. Most healers, as will be discussed later, acquire their skills by apprenticeship or by spiritual inspiration. However, healers are reluctant to divulge their secrets and many die without ever choosing an apprentice.

The central reasons for the secrecy surrounding healing knowledge are: (1) healing skills represent power; and power of one sort or another is necessary for gaining a name – thus some have chiefly power and others have medicines. A person seeking to accrue power will not want to divide his power too soon by taking an apprentice. Rather, he will build his name on the merits of his healing and possibly, before he dies, share his learning. (2) To the Bariba, life consists of opposing forces. A person will try to acquire strength (*dam*: force, strength, power) but correspondingly, one can diminish one's amount by giving it away. In discussing the question of the power of healers, Mburu (1977) quoted a Nigerian herbalist who explained:

It is the way herbal medicine is mixed and used that varies from one doctor to another, the best being the one who has his own way of mixing herbs in such a way that the result is more effective than another. That is the specialist. He will not be eager to reveal this special expertise. *He stops being a specialist when he has no special knowledge.* (my italics)

(3) Medicines are, in the words of one healer, a serious matter. One cannot give knowledge regarding medicines, their collection, preparation, or administration to just anyone; giving medicines to a young person is a mark of great confidence. Others may say that medicines should not be given to the young, or the old will kill them from envy. One healer told a European priest disapprovingly that whites give knowledge to anyone and would do well to be more guarded. (4) Knowledge of medicines cannot be given easily; a responsible healer must know the character and motivation of the person who is seeking to learn from him. Whether a healer decides to share his knowledge with another depends on whether the seeker wants to know for reasons of conceit, for self-interest, or to make good use. One well-known healer said that in his life, he has never used medicines for evil, but many have come to ask for medicines for maleficent purposes. When a person arrives requesting knowledge, he discusses the issue at length with the person until he can sense if the man is "strong, patient and can pardon." Because the supplicant rarely possesses those characteristics, the healer will give him false information. For example, if a medicine requires substances from seven trees, the healer will cite five names so that the supplicant will go away content and not wish him harm but the medicines will be useless or weak. A healer, then, will treat others regardless of their strength of character but will not explain the treatment.

In answer to the question "why do some people have medicines whereas others have none?" a group discussion elicited the response that a person needs to have an old person as a teacher. Old people do not do this until they are *very* old and they may die without showing anyone their medicine. If this happens, the young will regret their loss greatly. Does this mean that a person with no elderly healer in the family, or a person whose powerful relative dies close-mouthed, can never become knowledgeable? The consensus was no, an individual can leave his residence and kin and go to "another place" where one can pay to learn medicines. If one goes to such a place, the residents will teach the apprentice for a fee willingly because they know the apprentice will eventually leave and take his knowledge elsewhere to apply it.

I personally found this philosophy to be evident in that some healers were willing to give me medicines and/or information because they thought that I would soon leave to practice my skills far away and could not be considered competition. Thus Mburu suggested:

In very many respects, the African traditional doctor is more at home with foreigners because he erroneously considers them ignorant of his modus operandi and modus vivendi. The white person is a temporary visitor without any interests ... the fellow native is a threat to the traditional practitioners (158).

A Bariba apprentice who learns by leaving his residence and heading for a distant region will not divulge his learning but many praise the name and wisdom of the one who taught him, especially if that person is far away. The place name where the apprenticeship was served may also be extolled, as in the song of Bori, a village located about 175 kilometers from Pehunko and renowned for its powerful healers. Musicians often sing the song, accompanied by a three-stringed guitar:

The Song of the Medicines of Bori

Tim do m kom sɛ̃ An tim kĩkpa bori da bori gibu tim do mɛkom sɛ̃ an bori gibu tim kĩkpa tam dɛri an tam dɛri kpa kurɔ dɛri an bori gibu tim kĩkpa kurɔ dɛri	The medicines are good but difficult to make. If you want medicines, go to Bori. Bori people's medicines are good but difficult. If you want their medicine, leave drink alone; if you leave drink and leave women, if you want the Bori medicines, leave women alone (while learning.)

5.1.2. *Apprenticeship*

Although most healers claim to have acquired at least part of their knowledge from another healer, by occasional observation or by lengthy apprenticeship, some use of medicines (substances) and words may be learned from spiritual sources. Non-human sources may include voices which speak to the individual in question during the night without any corporeal presence evident, dreams, and special mystical encounters. Usually spirits only come in dreams *after* the individual possesses a spirit (e.g., has spirit cult membership) or has been involved with a spirit. One such possible route to healing wisdom is "*toora*." "*Toora*" refers to the tiny, "different" leaves which are infrequently seen to be growing on the top of a high tree. A person who sees these leaves (e.g., red, matchlike flowers at the upper foliage of an orange tree) has the option of deciding to spend the night under the tree. During the night, terrifying visions of animals and monsters will appear, transformed from the "*toora*" leaves, and instruct the waiting apprentice. A person must be very brave to dare to spend the night in the bush and to encounter these frightening apparitions, but the reward is knowledge of substances useful in curing, and increment of "power."

In principle, a medicine person can turn medicines for good or evil; thus " . . . the person who knows the cure, knows the poison and the curse too" (Mburu 1977:172). Similarly, Bariba say that a person did so much evil that he can't heal anymore. In spite of the potential for doing harm, however, there is a definite distinction between a medicine person and a poisoner (*dobo*) who does only harm. A medicine person is also called *baaba*, (father) because he is like a master, or a father. In referring to a healer then, a person might say "*oo, baa wa*," "he is a master," meaning that he has many medicines. Few terms exist in Bariba for differentiating types of healers, other than "tamabu," a clan name which includes reference to those people who heal sprains, breaks, and muscle complaints.

Otherwise, healers who treat disorders ranging from hemorroids to abcesses, coughs, childhood illnesses, and insanity are all known as medicine people (*tingibu*).

One distinction that should be made, however, is that between a medicine person and a diviner. This categorization is discussed by Mburu who believes that the dichotomy between "herbalist" and "diviner" is Africa-wide. Although Mburu uses the term herbalist, the characterization of the position suggests that the equivalent is the Bariba "medicine person." An herbalist, according to Mburu, " . . . literally, is a person who deals with herbs and herbal medicines of whatever brand concoted from selected leaves, roots or any other properties of plants. The medication thereof is explicitly for specific diseases not their underlying supernatural cause. The herbalist has the modern pharmacist as a counterpart in modern medicine." (169) Empirical knowledge of herbs, then, is the main requisite.

A diviner, on the other hand, "is the religious-medical specialist who not only defines illness but also divines the circumstances of the illness. He gives the *ultimate* etiological conditions of a psychic, somatic or psycho-somatic disorder, interpersonal alliances, and conflicts." (Mburu 1977: 169) Healing, he concludes, is one thing, divining another, and a patient may need one, another, or both. Data on the Bariba certainly supports this conclusion. Nonetheless, it is necessary to remark that there is a great deal of overlap among "medicine people" and diviners among the Bariba. The overlap occurs in that many diviners (*sɔrɔ*) are also medicine people but the reverse is much less often true. When referring to a medicine person, then, I am not referring to a specialist who deals with questions of ultimate causation, but who handles simple diagnosis and treatment. Diviners will be specifically referred to as such.

Another proviso is that "medicine" does not refer to substances used for simple ailments such as colds or minor diarrhea; every Bariba possesses some such knowledge, but is not considered a medicine person. A medicine person is one who possesses cures for serious complaints which require complicated cures and cures with strength or power. The definition of medicine held by the Bariba corresponds generally to that suggested by Glick, who defined medicine as "any substance used as part of a response to illness in the expectation that some of its power will augement that of the patient" (Glick 1967:38).

Bariba cures may comprise a combination of substances such as leaves, roots, animal parts, and words. In fact, it is the knowledge of words which distinguishes the layperson from the specialist.

5.1.3. *The Power of Words*

Knowledge of special words which carry the power to heal or harm is a characteristic of a true healer. Many Bariba know a few such words or incantations, but the sign of a specialist is the possession of more incantations than the ordinary Bariba has available, and these carry particular weight. Incantations are often inherited by a person from a relative but may be altered slightly by the user. Often an incantation accompanies the use of a medicine and the incantation requests the desired effect of the medicine. The significance of the power of words to Bariba should not be underestimated. When attempting to unravel the complex associations of substances and words used in curing, the western researcher might be tempted to focus on botanical substances ingested or otherwise applied to the body of the sick person. To the Bariba, however, knowledge of a substance may be much less meaningful than possession of incantations. As one woman explained it, everyone knows some leaves or bark or roots which cure. But a true healer knows the words to say before cutting the substance and again, before putting the substance in the pot (while collecting). The speaking of special words is indicative of the potential potency of the treatment.

As a general aside on the power of words, it is interesting to consider the example of the word *daura. Daura* came to my attention as a word sung in the Bariba death chant of the pure (commoner) Bariba. A young, French-speaking Bariba translated this phrase as "*daura worama* . . . a heavy sound, like the sound of a tree falling, or the force of the wind felling a tree." Another explanation was that if the chief dies and you come bearing the news, you will die if you report the news before the drums beat, so instead of saying "the chief is dead," you report "*daura worama*" and everyone understands. Later, I decided to verify this interpretation with the *gooyankuko*, the woman who leads the death chants at a funeral. This ritual specialist refused to even repeat the words or to explain the meaning, claiming that *daura* refers to death; the word itself is the essence of death, and that it was not good to say it (perhaps at an inappropriate occasion, e.g., not a funeral).

Similarly, Kamuti Kiteme, (Grolling 1976) writing on "Traditional African Medicine" states that African healers administer medicines orally but also instruct patients to wear "curative objects" (414) whose "healing effects" are controlled by the healer. It is not the object itself that is powerful . . . "actually, the procedure is . . . related to the POWER OF THE WORD from a doctor's mouth. The doctor's 'word' is more powerful than the medicine itself. And so he can, at any time, change the healing power of any given object to treat totally different diseases successfully . . . " It is the power of the word which allows the substance to meet different needs, depending on the requirements of the situation.

5.1.4. *Midwife as Healer*

The midwife *may* be a medicine person, respected for her power, or she may merely be a "person who assists at deliveries," who may claim knowledge of a few more medicines than the average woman but the range of her skills and knowledge does not afford her the recognition of being powerful. One would not say of such a midwife, "she has force," (*dam*). To a man, *dam* is represented in terms of children, women, crops, political power, healing power, and in contemporary times, money. To a woman, healing knowledge is the major non-ascribed form of authority and power other than the ability to commune with spirits, a capacity which some midwives possess. Female healers, then, may transcend the boundaries of sex, particularly when menopausal, and achieve a degree of power and influence which no woman holds in the public domain.

One approach to analyzing the meaning of the role and status of the midwife is through the terminology for the function which she serves. Names and titles are highly significant to Bariba, as is demonstrated in the elaborate and ritualized salutation procedure and in the institution of praise-singing. In most social interactions, name translates status. Names are especially linked to status in the form of aristocratic titles but are also indicative in referring to occupation, especially in the cases where occupation is in correlation with clan.

5.1.5. *Midwifery as a Category*

The Bariba midwife is not referred to by a special title. She is addressed by clients as "mother" as are all older women by younger women; by her age cohorts she will be addressed either by name or by the term *berɛ* (older sister) as respect dictates in the particular encounter. In describing a birth assistant, a person may say:

u ra maru si wa (from maru, delivery; si, to do)	she is (habitually) one who does deliveries

However, *marusio* cannot be considered as an occupational category comparable either to the major occupational categories offered by Bariba themselves as significant classifications, or to other titles referred to in greetings.

Two points of significance regarding the terms of reference for a midwife are (1) praises are rarely sung for women, other than for the few women who serve official functions such as the chief's sister, the Yɔ̃ Kogi. Contrastingly, male notables have praise names and special phrases which are drummed and chanted for them and by which they can be recognized by other local Bariba. (2) *Marusio* is not a term comparable to blacksmith or butcher in that it does not encompass descent and occupation; in other words, midwifery is not comprised in one of the clan names which refer to hereditary occupations and which serve as praise names, although midwifery is a skill which is usually transmitted through family members, often through patrilineal kin. Bariba distinguish midwifery from hereditary occupations by saying that it is not *bwɛsɛru*. This word might loosely be translated as "family" and refers usually to patrilineal kin but also can apply to matrilineal kin, within the range of which exact links may not necessarily be known.

Midwifery, then, is not considered as a family occupation, but rather, as an idiosyncratic skill, more to be compared to carpentry (in that one may have a talent and an interest in it) than smithing or circumcising. As a skill, midwifery fits into the larger category of healing. A midwife who is respected as a healer might accordingly be praised and addressed as "medicine person," as follows:

Salutation	fɔ mako	Greeting *clan name*
Reply	mm	Acknowledgement
Salutation	fɔ *tingi*	Greetings *medicine person*

It is important to note, though, that although some midwives are healers, others would not be considered in this frame of reference. This distinction will be discussed and illustrated in the following section focusing on social characteristics of Bariba midwives.

5.2. IMPLICATIONS OF ROLE EXPECTATIONS FOR BIRTH ASSISTANCE

Expectations regarding the attributes of the midwife, such as training or socio-economic status serve as significant considerations in the selection of a birth attendant. These sociological and career attributes include: religion, age, residence, education, marital and family status, recruitment, apprenticeship, remuneration, role variability, and spirit possession. The particular topics were selected either because they are standard sociological variables, used here as guidelines to eliciting significant features of the midwife, or because they were believed to be salient in Bariba culture and hence likely to be revelant in client-practitioner interactions. Such items are detailed in the text.

These attributes, then, will be delineated and examined in order to outline the characteristics of the typical Bariba midwife and to discuss the hypothesis that in order to fulfill role expectations, the midwife must demonstrate attributes which fall within an acceptable range to the client population, thus rendering her reasonably homophilous. Homophily, as defined in Chapter 1, is "the degree to which pairs of individuals who interact are similar in certain attributes such as beliefs, values, education, social status and the like," (Rogers and Shoemaker 1971:200) whereas heterophily refers to the degree to which individuals who interact differ in certain attributes.

As suggested in Chapter 1, a healer (in this instance, a midwife) is selected in order to accomplish a particular task; a client assumes certain characteristics of the role occupant are requisite for the healer to be effective and competent. Clients and indigenous midwives are found to be homophilous in that they share concepts of causation, beliefs, values, and role expectations. This is not to argue that homophily refers to shared social status but that the midwife and her clients share expectations on the attributes of a midwife, how to relate to one another, on diagnosis, techniques and practices and goals. Chapters 6 and 7 will consider the implications of shared expectations regarding concepts of sickness causation, therapy techniques and practices. Here the emphasis will be on one aspect of role expectations – that regarding appropriate characteristics of the role occupant. Contrastingly, where the healer is not homophilous with the client, as will be shown to be the case, the absence of homophily operates to deter prospective clients from utilizing obstetrical services. Thus in the case of the nurse-midwife/client relationship, the respective role occupants will be shown not to be homophilous. In contrast to the indigenous midwife, the nurse-midwife does not share significant attributes, values and expectations with her client and this lack of homophily deters clients from selecting the nurse-midwife as an option for birth assistance.

5.2.1. *Status Characteristics of Midwives*

Cosminsky notes that many ethnographic reports do not differentiate a specialized status of midwife from any birth attendant. (In addition, the World Health Organization also classifies together all birth attendants as "traditional birth attendants" if they assist at deliveries but have no 'formal' training.) Cosminsky, then, uses the term midwife in reference to "a position which has been socially differentiated as a specialized status by the society. Such a person is usually regarded as a specialist and a professional in her own eyes and by her community" (Cosminsky 1976:231). Differentiating a "birth attendant" from a midwife is not always simple, however, and even a differentiated status such as the Bariba *marusio* (person who does deliveries) can include persons demonstrating widely varying degrees of capability and types of powers. Thus some midwives are healers, others are noted for a more purely technical skill but in this study all are differentiated definitionally from a birth attendant such as a female relative who may be present at delivery and merely support the parturient from behind while she is kneeling in labor.

Henceforth, indigenous midwives will be referred to by the French term which is used locally – matrones – in order to avoid confusion with government midwives.

Initially, at the onset of the study, names of ten area matrones were obtained from the Mayor of Pehunko. These matrones had volunteered to participate several months previously in a Ministry of Health Training program for indigenous midwives which had not in fact been held. The additional matrones came to my attention through interviews with officials in surrounding villages and through informants throughout the district. The total number of matrones in the district of Kouande has not been determined and efforts to do a census of matrones was not considered to be worth the logistical problems and time input compared to the benefits of more intensive interviewing of fewer matrones. However, the matrones interviewed do include the most well-known matrones in the prominent villages of the district and most well-known matrones in the Commune of Pehunko are included in the sample.

5.2.1.1. *Religion*

Of the 18 matrones, 6 were Muslim, 11 animist, and one claimed to be Muslim but participated in Bariba spirit possession cult ceremonies addressing earth spirits and was respected for her knowledgeability regarding customary beliefs and practices. Religion was originally expected to be a significant variable because of the cultural differences between non-Muslim and Muslim Bariba but does not seem to be significant in terms of delivery procedures. It also seemed possible that clients might prefer matrones to government midwives because of "religious" similarities between the client and birth attendant but the data did not suggest this factor to be relevant.

5.2.1.2. *Age*

As is shown in Table 2 all matrones except one were postmenopausal; 83% of those interviewed were over age 50 and all were 40 or older.

TABLE 2
Matrones by age

	Under 30	30–40	40–50	50–60	Over 60
No.	0	0	3	5	10
%	0	0	17	28	56

5.2.1.3. *Birth and Residence*

This question was considered potentially significant because of implications for matrone-client relationships based on genealogical ties; e.g., in the instance of patrilocal residence and marriage in the same village, clients might be selected from patrilineal kin. In actuality, approximately 1/3 of those who responded were not living in the village where they were born or grew up (see Table 3). However, the question of links with kin was not pursued due to great reluctance on the part of the matrones to discuss kinship linkages. Further investigation regarding clients of matrones suggested that although matrones do serve kin, selection of a matrone is likely to be on a neighborhood basis.

TABLE 3
Birth and residence locations of matrones

	Currently residing in birthplace	Residing elsewhere	No answer	Residing with brother
No.	4	6	7	1
%	22	33	39	6

5.2.1.4. *Education*

Because most rural Bariba women have received no formal education, it was assumed that matrones would similarly have no formal educational background and that this lack of formal education would contribute to homophily between matrones and clients. As predicted, of the 18 matrones, 17 had no education whatsoever and could not speak French or read or write in either French or

Bariba. One matrone residing in Pehunko center had three years of schooling, beginning in 1919. She had retained some knowledge of spoken French; her comprehension was good but her speaking ability less fluent. She could not currently read or write. This matrone had also traveled to the capital, Cotonou, and had acquired a stock of stories and observations about other ethnic groups which accorded her a reputation for being somewhat more cosmopolitan than most of her age contemporaries, other than a few female traders and "*El Hadjiyas*" who had been to Mecca.

5.2.1.5. *Marital Status*

Marital status was investigated in this survey in order to draw conclusions regarding the similarity of matrones in this respect to their clients, most of whom are married and also regarding possible conflicts between role responsibilities as a wife and as a professional.

TABLE 4
Marital status of matrones

	Unmarried	Currently married	Widow	Currently divorced	N.A.
No.	0	10	7	0	1
%	0	56	39	0	6

All those 17 matrones who responded had been married at one time; of those, over half were currently married. However, unlike the midwives described by Paul (1975), the fact of being married for these women is unlikely to entail responsibilities which must be disavowed in order to engage in the practice of midwifery. Also in contrast to the Mayan midwives, Bariba matrones in general are not obliged to "give up" or refuse sexual relations with their husbands because all except one are menopausal, and menopausal women cease sexual relations, according to Bariba tradition. Sexual relations can, in principle, affect the power of some medicines to work effectively and for men, who continue to have sexual relations with younger women, the prospect of certain rituals or healing practices may entail sexual abstinence for a variable period. Women are prohibited from handling potent medicines during menstruation because menstrual pollution may "kill" the essence of the medicine. This proscription is often extended to cover a woman during the entirely of her reproductive years so that a woman cannot prepare or use powerful medicines until she has ceased menstruating, at which time she becomes "like a man." Given the many years "head start" of men, who have occasion to experiment with medicines from adolescence, it is the rare woman who can claim to complete with a man in terms of healing knowledge and skills. A woman may, however, be apprenticed during her pre-menopausal years, during which time she accumulates information. Some women may, in fact learn from their husbands. In this sample of matrones, three acquired the basis of their knowledge from their husbands; two of these husbands were particularly noted for their prowess and one husband was a diviner as well as a healer. These wives learned from their husbands when both spouses were elderly; this is perhaps related to the generally held suspicion and mistrust with which "wives" are held, due to the assumption that a wife never really belongs to her husband's family and the expectation that at some point in time, she may decide to leave her husband and go home, taking her knowledge with her to her own kin.

5.2.1.6. *Occupation of Husband*

This topic was investigated in order to determine whether similarities existed between the occupations of husbands of matrones and those of the clients and also whether matrones tended to be drawn from any particular social strata as indicated by marital alliance. Generally, the question was not very illuminating and produced only the information that of 17 respondents, 12 were wives of peasants, two of traders, and two others are the wives of former chiefs of the villages of Pehunko and Doh.

5.2.1.7. *Family Origin*

Although the 1972 revolution has prohibited traditional ethnic and class distinctions, these indices of identification continue to be recognized in rural areas such as the District of Kouande. The significant class distinctions include the *wasangari* (aristocrats), the *baatombu* (commoners and original settlers of the land), *gando* (slaves) and others such as Hausa, Yoruba, Djerma and Mossi immigrants. Although the Fulbe are considered a part of Bariba feudal society (Lombard 1965), I did not interview any Fulbe women because I did not speak Fulfulde and had problems maintaining informants both in Bariba villages and Fulbe camps. Therefore, I restricted my sample to women who considered themselves "Bariba" (both aristocrats and commoners) or some wives of Bariba men.

Of the matrones interviewed, six (33%) were aristocrats; ten (56%) commoners, one (6%) Hausa, and one identified herself as "*alifa*," or Muslim, with no other commentary. Husbands' family origins included seven aristocrats, seven commoners, one Hausa, one Nago and two unknown. Among these marriages there were only two between the traditional categories; that is, one aristocrat-commoner and one aristocrat-Hausa marriage. Marriage relationships were considered significant to this research because aristocratic and commoner rituals are sometimes quite different (baptism and funerals, for example); additionally, many more aristocrats have converted to Islam. It was suspected that husbands of different background might introduce their wives to new information and techniques, for example, "Words" taken from the Koran in the case of a Muslim spouse or a magic ring from an aristocratic family. Three matrones did in fact learn practices of different origin via their husbands; however, the cultural mix is probably much greater than this would suggest because of the number of matrones who learned medicines originally from a relative or mentor of different background.

5.3. RECRUITMENT OF MATRONES AND METHOD OF SKILL ACQUISITION

Matrones were interviewed regarding recruitment and method of skill acquisition in order to draw conclusions regarding the uniformity in recruitment and training of matrones, on midwifery as a family specialty, and on variance among matrones in type of training and source of skill acquisition.

In casual conversation, Bariba women claimed that skills such as midwifery were learned from a woman's mother. However, the matrones in this sample did not tend to have learned midwifery from a "true" mother; only 4/18 (22%) had done so. Rather, the recruitment pattern varied as is shown in Table 5. Fifty-six per cent of the matrones claimed some relative was a matrone; six said no relative was ever a matrone, and one did not respond. Matrones most commonly learned midwifery from a grandmother or mother. These patterns are congruent with the patterns of child socialization customary to Bariba.

TABLE 5
Matrone recruitment patterns

grandmother										
fa mo	?	momo	mo	husb mo	god	fa sis	husband	spirits	n.a.
2	1	2	4	3	2	1	1	1	1

Seventy-two per cent of the matrones claimed to have learned midwifery by means of an apprenticeship. Most described the process of learning as "observation," ("I watched her . . . ") or "carrying the *calebasse*" for an established matrone. ("Carrying the *calebasse*" refers to the apprentice accompanying the matrone and carrying her medicine gourd and vials for her.) Two others learned by divine blessing, one from dreams, one from experiment and practice, and one preferred not to explain. With regard to the belief evidenced by Bariba women that midwifery is learned from one's mother, two matrones mentioned the *expectation* among neighbors and kin that if one's mother was a matrone, her daughter will be equally knowledgeable. Yaayi Karami Okpe gave her account of such a situation saying that she had lived with her mother but never really watched her work or bothered to ask questions. When her mother died, people came to her because her mother had helped them. She would tell those who asked for her help that she didn't know anything, but they would reply, "you lived with her, you just are not a good person, you don't want to help." So she began to assist at deliveries, and when problems arose, she would ask "an older person" about appropriate measures to take, then she experimented a bit on her own, and now she is competent.

In other cases of interest, Yaayi Gingire, as a little girl, observed her maternal grandmother. Her mother's brother Dogi who was approximately 15 years older than she, also was very interested in healing knowledge and the two of them followed the grandmother together. Later, Dogi became a famed healer and taught Gingire himself. Dogi recently died but Gingire knows many of his medicines. Gingire pointed out that one can observe and assist a grandmother but many years may pass before one can practice alone. Although three matrones learned from their husband's mothers, matrones claim that it is unusual for such a relationship to develop. Thus Yaayi Yon Sika says "if you [the matrone] are away, people come and ask for your daughter, thinking she has seen you. No one comes to ask for your son's wife." Others say that it is imprudent to divulge information to a son's wife because no matter how long she has lived with her husband, she may leave and return to her own kin. The exception to this which would allow a matrone to teach her son's wife is "when there is love between you." Yaayi Ganigi, who learned from her husband's mother, described her learning as follows: "my husband's mother washed the child and I watched her. When she was old, she told me to do it. She told me to help the woman and stay by her for seven days [to wash the newborn] and I did." In order to increase her understanding of medicines, throughout the years, she has asked several old men for information on how to cure more successfully.

One way of understanding recruitment of matrones is to examine the prospective replacements of the matrones. To this end, I asked the matrones in this sample, "will your daughter be a matrone," and if not, "who are you teaching or planning to teach?" Only 4 of 14 matrones who responded were planning to have a daughter as an apprentice; of the others who planned to take an apprentice, the choices included a sister's daughter (1), brother's daughter (2), granddaughter (1) and younger sister (1). One other replied that her brother's daughter would replace her, and one that she would teach her granddaughter. Yaayi Yon Sika expressed the alternatives most succinctly:

> If you had a choice between your own child, your brother's daughter, or your son's wife, who would you choose? You would choose your own daughter or your brother or sister's daughter, not your son's wife – she is from elsewhere and will return there. You may also show your granddaughter if she is clever.

According to this matrone, any daughter may learn regardless of her rank among children; the choice depends on the courage, charitability and resourcefulness of the daughter. In her case, it is her son who has expressed an interest in learning, whereas her daughters have not. For this disinterest she has chastized them, reminding them that if she dies, people will come to ask them for help and none of them will know anything useful.

Several matrones claimed that the Bariba "way" is for a grandmother to teach her granddaughter; as was pointed out previously, 5/18 of the matrones in this sample learned from their grandmothers, but only one plans to teach her granddaughter. Most of the matrones explained that they were not yet ready to take an apprentice, although all except two were over 50 years of age. Four of the 14 matrones who discussed this issue stated that they would *never* take an apprentice, but the others claimed that they were not ready yet or the apprentice was too young. According to this matrone, one's own or sister's daughter is the most likely apprentice; the more courageous she is, the younger she can begin to assist at deliveries. Correspondingly, one matrone said she hasn't found anyone courageous to replace her yet, whereas another is blind now and never got around to showing her daughters or nieces who were interested. One matrone who learned from her husband explained that she isn't planning to pass on her knowledge because she is successful by means of involving her husband's name together with other special words; these words cannot be transmitted to an apprentice.

A matrone who claimed to have learned from spirits in dreams said she won't ever tell anyone what she knows or the spirits will leave her in anger. Finally, Gingire, the matrone who learned from her grandmother, together with her mother's brother Dogi who became famed throughout the region, said she plans to teach Dogi's daughter because Dogi had started to do so himself before he died.[17] In sum, only four matrones were actively involved in teaching an apprentice; of these, one was teaching her sister, one her sister's daughter, one her brother's daughter, and one her own youngest daughter.

5.4. SOURCES OF MEDICAL KNOWLEDGE

When asked to specify the source of their healing knowledge, eleven matrones described an apprenticeship, three said they learned from spirits in dreams, one solicited information periodically from an elder, one said she experimented primarily on her own, and one said it wasn't any concern of the researcher. One matrone said, speaking generally, that if a woman is competent and her mother or grandmother was a matrone, she is a suitable and likely successor to the position. This response fits the data most accurately. Other matrones, in discussing recruitment to the position of matrone, offered a variety of responses, usually based on their own experience, except for one who said that no matter who one learns from, God is involved. Regarding the question of those who claimed to learn from dreams and/or spirits, I asked both those who gave such a response and those who learned from another human healer to comment on how this type of learning was transmitted. The ones who learned from spirits said that they heard voices, usually in the night, but saw no one. The voices explained how to deal with certain problems, or what substances to prepare for curing.

Some matrones who had learned from a healer said that even if a matrone claimed to have learned only from spirits, she really had learned from a person as well. A consideration of curing procedures in general suggests, though, that while the matrones may in fact have learned from a human being, dreams are frequently evoked by healers as modes of transmission of information. Thus one healer treats childhood illnesses by listening to a description of the complaint and telling the parent to return the following day with a pot. During the night, the healer will have collected the substance (usually leaves, roots, bark) and will put them in the pot. Another healer remarked that dreams sometimes reveal which of the leaves or roots or other substances one knows would be successful in treating a certain complaint. In other words, in dreams, the healer's existing knowledge is synthesized and "experiments" are suggested for trial. It was not clear whether spirits are believed to have any function in transmitting these dreams or producing the voices although one matrone implied that spirits are responsible for dream revelations.

5.5. MATRONES OWN REPRODUCTIVE HISTORIES

Interest in the question of number of pregnancies and living children derived from beliefs regarding mothers whose children always die. The Bariba express great concern over these children and the reasons for this misfortune, which might be related to sorcery, witchcraft, or merely to destiny. It seemed likely that a mother afflicted by consistent infant or child mortality or a woman who suffered the supreme misfortune of never conceiving or always aborting would not be a desirable candidate to become a matrone, due to the possibility of passing on the bad luck, harming a client through envy, or somehow involving a third party in her own misfortune.

Matrones tended to feel that questions regarding their families were intrusive and irrelevant, therefore five refused to answer and no information was acquired on them. Information on the others was obtained in part from the matrones and in part from other villagers. Of the 13 matrones on whom data were obtained, all had experienced two or more pregnancies and all had at least two living children. The relationship between number of pregnancies and number of living children is shown in Table 6.

Although the information on reproductive histories of matrones is very sketchy, and the sample is small, a rough comparison between the proportion of live births ending in infant or child death among women over 40 in the general population and among matrones suggests that possibly matrones have suffered a lower rate of loss.[18] These reproductive histories of good fortune may contribute to success of matrones in the practice of midwifery. What is certain is that a woman who has no pregnancies or no living children would be most unlikely either to be recruited as a matrone or to attract a clientele.

5.6. AGE AT UNSUPERVISED DELIVERY

The discussion of apprenticeship suggested that young women were not appropriate apprentices; thus one matrone indicated her three daughters, ranging in age from 35 to 20 and said all were too young to discuss medicines. Correspondingly,

TABLE 6
Reproductive histories of thirteen matrones

No. pregnancies	Living children
2	2
3+	3
3+	3+
4	?
3+	3+
2	2
?	2
7	3
5	3+
3	3
7	7
12	6
4+	4

most matrones claimed to have been menopausal or post-menopausal before assisting at an unsupervised delivery. Two matrones demurred, saying that neither was menopausal when she began practicing alone.

5.7. ASSISTANCE AT OWN CHILD'S DELIVERY

The topic of a matrone's assistance at her own child's delivery was addressed because of the cultural norms idealizing modesty between a mother and daughter; propriety inhibits an adult woman from displaying her genitals in her mother's presence. Although mothers in general attended a daughter's delivery more often than would be expected given verbalizations on the subject (see Chapter 7), most matrones did not do so.[19]

Of eleven matrones with whom this issue was discussed, three said they definitely would assist at a daughter's delivery, one stating the equivalent of "charity begins at home." Seven matrones said it was improper to treat one's own daughter, and one said she would give advice and suggest medicines but would not be physically present in the room with her daughter. Correspondingly, most women of reproductive age stated that it would be very rare to have one's "own" mother present at a delivery, in fact it would be embarrassing and improper and a women would "eat shame" to have her mother see her nakedness.

5.8. REMUNERATION

Matrones were interviewed regarding remuneration as part of a more general effort to elicit information on the social position of the matrone and on midwifery as a specialty in comparison to other specialties. Remuneration, respect and other indicators of gratitude, were considered to be indicative of the value attributed to the role of matrone and hence to have implications for selection of birth assistance.

Midwifery is a part-time specialty, closest in comparability to artisan specialties but not bringing in the cash income of other part-time specialties which are in the "modern" sphere such as barbering, photography or shoe repair. Midwifery as a part-time specialty which does not necessarily bring in a dependable income is not comparable to any of the full-time occupations such as carpentry or repairwork. A few matrones sell medicines on the side in the market, especially for the common woman's complaint "*tigpiru*" but this is a more commerical side than is usually evidenced by matrones regarding their midwifery skills.

As women, they do engage in activities for financial gain but these enterprises are seen as primarily economic, and distinct from midwifery. Almost all Bariba women engage in some commercial activities in order to obtain a cash income. Perhaps the most common enterprises are prepared-food vending and what is referred to locally as "small trading," that is, selling of a variety of items such as cigarettes, candy, sugar, canned tomato paste, combs, soap, hair plaiting, thread, etc. Matrones engaged in a variety of commercial activities ranging from sales of kola nuts, cotton thread, small trading, to preparation and sales of millet beer or distilled liquor. However, income from healing does not seem to represent a significant portion of revenue for most matrones and midwifery should not be considered an "occupation" in the sense of an activity which brings in regular remuneration. In contemporary times, matrones may receive both money and produce or cloths in return for their services. However, remuneration is variable and very much dependent on the will, or charitability, or the clients and their families. Many matrones, when asked about payment for services, remarked in disgust that "some people forget what they owe you so quickly that they neglect to say good-morning the next day." A salutation may be the only recompense a matrone receives for preparing and administering medicines, and assisting at a delivery.

When do they receive payment for services, matrones receive such goods as butter, soap, oil, 2 meters of cloth, produce (rarely); some matrones claim that they don't accept gifts from clients, only salutations while others don't accept payment from family. This latter condition raises interesting possibilities in the village of Doh, where most villagers are related and a matrone could clearly not expect to earn much income from providing medicines and assisting at births. Baby washers (whether birth assistants or not) receive the most standardized payment – usually a hunk off the soap prepared for the new baby and porridge and sauce. In Pehunko, with its large Muslim population, one finds Muslim families who kill a sheep for a new baby's baptism on the eight day after birth; the sheep is divided among dignitaries in a predetermined fashion and the baby washer receives her special part, the neck. In such families, however, if a matrone assisted at the delivery, but was not the baby washer, she may not receive a portion of the meat. It seems, then, that a matrone accrues prestige and respect for her healing activities, rather than financial gain.

Cosminsky, in her review "Cross-Cultural Perspectives on Midwifery"

(Cosminsky 1976) stated that the midwife usually occupies a respected position but her status is not invariably a high one. The indigenous midwife in India, to list one instance, is held in low esteem due to beliefs regarding pollution. In considering the status of the Bariba matrone, one finds examples of some customary modes of indicating respect such as praise-singing (for the greatly admired), and reference by the title "medicine person," which suggest a high status for the matrone.

Genuflexion is also an indication of the degree of respect with which one person perceives another. A matrone would certainly receive a deep genuflexion from a client following some assistance. Confusion may arise in interpreting this gesture, however, because a younger person always should bow deeply to an elder and it is necessary to establish which aspect of the social identity of the matrone has received deference.[20] Nonetheless, those matrones known for their competence and esoteric knowledge are seen to receive full genuflexions (in which the person of lesser status squats on the ground rather than merely dipping the knees) from women, men and other elderly people. When one elderly person meets a matrone and genuflects deeply, indicating lower status in the relationship in this manner, clearly prestige rather than age is at issue.

Gifts are an important indicator of position in Bariba society; a tribute system was intrinsic to the traditional feudal social organization. However, gift-giving was found not to form an obligatory aspect of the client-practitioner interaction. It seems rather that a healer with many substances to dispense in curing, and knowledge of incantations to provide potency to the treatments, increases his prestige by not accepting or requiring payment, so that the populace is always in the healer's debt, and in obligation to the healer's charity and goodwill. Some matrones did state that although they are irregularly paid at the time of delivery assistance, clients or their relatives may present gifts such as butter or mustard or yams on feast occasions to show gratitude and admiration. Other comparative aspects of the tribute system were difficult to research due to the revolutionary doctrine prohibiting payment of tribute to any traditional functionaries. This prohibition particularly applied to political officials such as chiefs but it would have been interesting to observe the contrasts in types of gifts and tributes for the various statuses, whether political, service or craft positions.

Another minor indicator of respect often provided to the matrone is the salutation "*ka faaba*," (thank you for saving me) offered after a successful delivery, as well as the salutation "*ka tɔnu*," (thank you for a goodness done to a person). The fact that ordinary nonspecialists owe deference to the matrone is also evident in situations where the matrone arrives at a delivery and all other attendants leave. This is explained as behavior required to signify respect for the matrone's skills, which should not be observed by others for they are secret and should only be shared at the matrone's expressed wish. Retiring from a situation due to deference is characteristic of behavior of any person who finds him/herself surpassed in competence, whether it is a question of a layperson who calls a matrone, or a matrone who defers to a more skilled healer. Thus one matrone stated that she could not describe what another more powerful healer had done at a delivery because she had left, feeling "small," and not wanting to observe a superior at work. One must also remark the implicit flattery and esteem accorded to any person with powers of the occult and control over substances, whether this power is used for good or evil.

In analyzing the status of the matrone, and considering status in terms of the rights and duties associated with the position, it seems evident that the transaction between the matrone and her client is characterized by the offering of a service by the matrone which involves the mobilization of certain strengths (referred to earlier) as well as special skills and knowledge. In return for providing the capability and willingness to perform the role, the client is expected to reciprocate with deference and respect and gifts, but the last optionally. It is also possible that prior to the colonial era, when the customary statuses and roles were more in evidence and one could observe an individual's behavior in many contexts, one might have determined other significant indicators of a social identity. Currently, it is very difficult to compare the position of the midwife – respect to which she has claim, services or gifts which she receives – with that of other specialists and functionaries because public enactment of their roles has been greatly reduced. The literature is of little enlightenment on this issue because it deals almost exclusively with political organization and the roles of men; the most suggestive statement regarding prestige of women is that previously quoted wherein Lombard remarks that matrones were among the most influential women in Bariba society and their fame sometimes extended throughout a region. Unfortunately, given the changes which have already occurred in social organization and the special limits on tribute (for example, no celebration of the traditional new year, when gifts were exchanged), prohibitions on "mystification," and on ritual performances, some specific aspects of the behavioral implications of the matrone's position and the matrone-client relationship must remain speculative.

5.9. COMPREHENSIVE CARE BY MATRONES

The matrone was found to provide *less* comprehensive care than expected with regard to areas of specialization covered in her practice. Matrones were expected to provide counseling and treatment in areas of specialization theoretically associated with reproduction; thus questioning revolved around those areas of health care, with which a specialist in women's problems might possibly deal. In interviews matrones were asked to describe the types of complaints they dealt with and they were questioned explicitly regarding the following subjects:

(1) menstrual problems;
(2) sterility;
(3) pregnancy and delivery;

(4) child care;
(5) nutrition;
(6) female circumcision.

Of 14 matrones who responded to these questions, none claimed competence in all the suggested areas; only two specialized in one single area. The most frequent response (6/14) was that the matrone's area of competence was pregnancy, childbirth and child care, particularly for children under three years of age. In this regard, Yaayi Yon Sika informed the researcher that any person who sought to assist women in childbirth needed to learn medicines for treating childhood ailments; these two facets of healing were logically associated. Two matrones, in addition to treating pregnant women and children, also dealt with other types of complaints; one with illnesses caused by sorcery and the other with common ailments of adults such as cough and stomach disorders. An additional matrone dealt with problems associated with pregnancy and delivery, child care, and menstrual complaints. One matrone specialized in "food counseling" for pregnant women with appetite problems during pregnancy. Two matrones handled pregnancy, child care and sterility problems and one of the latter also circumcised young girls. In sum, the "core" of the matrones activities was found to be delivery assistance, with some treatment of complaints associated with pregnancy such as appetite problems or preventive medicine for posible complications during labor.

5.10. PREGNANCY COUNSELING

The matrone's role does not usually include diagnosis of pregnancy. Women state that some primiparas need to consult a more knowledgeable woman in order to determine whether "it is a pregnancy or a sickness" but other women do not. Diagnosis of pregnancy, then, generally falls within the realm of every woman's competence. Most matrones can, however, tell if a woman is pregnant by observing the woman's breasts, skin color, general appearance, and of course, stomach size. Pregnancy diagnosis is considered a very private matter and one woman, who had experienced some ambiguous signs which she supposed might indicate either illness or pregnancy, said that she did not consult the matrone who delivered her last child, in order to diagnose her condition. Rather, she discussed her symptoms with an elderly woman in her husband's family in order to "keep the secrets of the household in the household." This statement might also indicate fear of sorcery against the unborn child by jealous outsiders.

The response to questions regarding treatment of sterility indicated the importance attached to this condition. Most matrones explained that treatment of sterility requires special knowledge and it is not everyone who is capable of dispensing such treatment. Sterility may be the result of several factors and before a cure can be attempted, an accurate diagnosis is required. Thus a person who treats sterility may be (but is not necessarily) a diviner or the afflicted person may consult a diviner first and then consult another specialist on sterility if the cause can be remedied by means of a healer's treatment. This type of recourse differs from that required if, for example, the cause of the sterility is a father's sister's curse. Overall, treatment of sterility necessitates special skills and powers not usually possessed by the matrone. The fact that one matrone functioned as a circumciser seems likely to be coincidence because female circumcision is a hereditary occupation, transmitted through women and was not found in this sample of matrones (with the one exception) to overlap with transmission of midwifery skills. Thus matrones remarked that female circumcision is *bweseru* ("family") but midwifery is not a hereditary speciality in the same sense.

The limited range of treatments offered by matrones corresponds to the general pattern of specialization of functions in Bariba culture, whether in the political sphere or in the domain of healing. Bariba healers include specialists for every common complaint. What seems to be significant is not range, but intensity of power. Thus it is more meaningful to be known as a medicine person than as a matrone.

5.11. MATRONE'S ROLE VARIABILITY

Within the domain of delivery and immediate post-partum assistance, the matrone's role is also variable. A matrone might serve the following functions:

(1) diagnose complications of labor;
(2) administer medicines for such complications;
(3) diagnose cause of retained placenta;
(4) cut the umbilical cord;
(5) administer medicines and apply remedies to expel the placenta;
(6) wash the baby;
(7) any combinations of the above.

Most matrones say that the primary distinction is between those who wash babies and those who do not; this division of labor is interpreted in various ways. One matrone claimed that women with "spirits on their heads" (that is, possession cult members) don't like to see blood or the placenta so they leave the scene of the delivery quickly; several village women suggested that baby washing is a fearful task to those with spirits; whereas others claim that those who wash babies need to have adequate time available and be skilled in the washing procedure in order to avoid causing the infant to be misshapen when older. This explanation implies that the reason for not washing babies is a lesser ability. However, all informants agree that although a specific skill may be required for the washing ritual, washers are not intrinsically as powerful as those matrones who assist at deliveries. That is, there are baby washers who do not assist at deliveries and who are not medicine people. There are also matrones who are medicine people, hence powerful, but who do not wash babies and some who do both. Of twelve matrones who discussed the range of their activities, half washed babies. Nine of those twelve cut the umbilical cord; the three who didn't claimed that a woman who is not protected by preventative medicines and who assists at a delivery and then stays to cut the cord, will go blind. This belief seemed fairly widespread, upon greater investigation, but no further explanation was forthcoming.

One baby washer who only cuts cords and washes but does not assist at complicated labors claimed that thirty years ago she washed all the babies in the village, even those of some now well-known matrones, but that now, "everyone" was taking on the job. Perhaps then, the division of labor is customary and the overlap is a relatively recent phenomenon.

5.12. SPIRIT POSSESSION

Approximately one-third of the matrones are adepts in spirit possession cults and of these, over 80% belong to the possession cult known as "*sambani*." Possession cults are characterized both by the types of spirits which possess the initiates and by the type of musical accompaniment to the possession dance. The two main cults are known as "*bukakaaru*" and "*sambani*;" *sambani* refers to a dance accompanied by gourd drums and rattles; *bukakaaru* includes musical accompaniment of gourd drums and guitars. Both sorts of cult are organized in associations led by a woman having attained her position by a combination of seniority[21] and prestige within the cult. *Bukakaaru* is a dance group of Djerma origin; the name of the spirit which possesses the women is known as "*bori*" (also found among Hausa). This spirit possesses women as they dance to the musical accompaniment. During the period of the dance, it is said that the possessed women no longer belong to their husbands. Instead, they have become the children of *kumba*, the cult leader and she alone can give them permission to return to their husbands. In the interim, the violinists may profit from the situation by forming liasons with the women, hence comes the saying that "if your wife is possessed by *bori*, she is the wife of the guitarists." (Evidently this applies to *sambani* adepts as well.)

Sambani, on the other hand, are possessed by spirits of the bush (*wɛrɛkugibu* or *bungibu*, the spirits of rocks, trees, streams, animals, etc.) The significant difference between the *bukakaaru* and *sambani* cult members is that *bukakaaru* adepts are possessed while dancing, and remember nothing afterwards. *Sambani*, in contrast, are noted for powers of clairvoyance, and the ability to read the future. Although *sambani* also cannot remember the possession event, they do retain the special powers of divination and clairvoyance remarked above. In this sense, *sambani* are alleged to be more powerful than *bukakaaru* adepts. Correspondingly, *bukakaaru* call *sambani* "husband," signifying that the status relationship between them resembles that of a wife respecting her spouse. In both *bukakaaru* and *sambani*, at the end of the initiation ceremony, before the initiate comes out of the trance, she is "taught" how to re-enter ordinary life

– cooking, cleaning, and other household activities are demonstrated as if she is entering a new life. In particular, she is re-introducted to sex and told "when you go to your husband and he touches you, don't scream. This happens to all women." Otherwise, it is said, he will touch her and she will scream and say "what's this? I have never heard of such a thing!" At the termination of the re-initiation to routine life, she is touched with a horse's tail and released from trance.

At that time, for *bukakaaru*, the extraordinary powers have ended. Some *bukakaaru* can foretell the future while possessed. One woman, for example, foretold the coming of a measles epidemic and suggested measures to weaken its virulence, but when not possessed, she is as limited in vision as a person who never "has spirits on her head," as possession is described. A *sambani*, on the other hand, can always throw cowrie shells or use other techniques of reading the future or divining the present. Of the matrones, all except one who had spirits on their heads were *sambani* adepts. The implication of *sambani* membership for a matrone will be discussed below.

It seemed of possible significance to determine whether matrones were selected from among women with spirits or whether, on the contrary, matrones tended to become cult members. This question proved very difficult to answer because the history of an individual's contact with spirits is perceived as extremely private. In fact, I obtained only three responses – two matrones were cult members before becoming matrones and the third became possessed after already being in practice. Regarding the frequency of spirit possession, not every household includes a woman who has spirits. (Men are rarely possessed, although one Pehunko male was known for the feats he had accomplished while undergoing initiation.) Some families, on the other hand, include several such women. Possession spirits are usually inherited, often from a father's sister or father's mother, although women claim that a cult member may bequeath her spirit to any well-loved relative. Spirits are usually inherited after death but are occasionally shared among the living, as in the case of a husband who shared his spirits with his wife.

At each of the two possession cult reunions which I attended, both of which were held to welcome new initiates, from 20–25 adepts were present and dancing. There appears to be a network of cult branches throughout the region. One group recently formed after splintering from a Pehunko-based membership; the cause of the split seems to have been a conflict over leadership occuring at the death of a cult superior. I was interested in possible links between a regional network of cults and members who are healers, but only a few healers seemed to have regional fame. In addition, only three spirit cults met during 1976–77, allegedly due to prohibitions on assemblies and on ritual drumming set forth by the national government. This restriction on cult activities rendered it difficult to estimate cult membership. Nonetheless, the small size of the two groups observed, which included Fulbe members, suggests a low frequency of possession among the population.

It seems likely that it is more than coincidence that one-third of the matrones are cult members and the majority of these are of the *sambani* variety. Cult membership provides contacts for a matrone to increase her knowledge about medicines, which may augment her diagnostic skills and inspire respect in her competence as a matrone. Moreover, both the role of matrone and that of spirit cult member seem to require certain similar character attributes, as will be detailed below.

5.13. INHERITANCE OF SPIRITS

A person may possess one or several spirits, each of which has a name. *Bukakaaru* members are all possessed by *bori* spirits but *sambani* members may be possessed by (1) *kiriku* spirits; (2) *biɔnkuro*; (3) *bunu*; (4) *wereku*. Each type of spirit has its own praises which the praise-singers chant to raise the spirit within its host but the women possessing different spirits can dance together because "all spirits are married with each other even as people marry amongst each other." Women are hierarchized according to the importance of what possessed them. For instance, a lion spirit is more important than a monkey. Relative prestige is indicated in praise-singing, musical accompaniment, money offered by spectators, etc.

If a person with spirits dies, the spirit may be bequeathed within the family or elsewhere. Some spirit possessors choose not to bequeath their spirits. In one case, a renowned healer had two types of spirits, *biɔnkuro* and *wereku*. The *wereku* are the spirits of other spirits, *wereku* of the bush, and can be very difficult to handle, causing illness or insanity. Accordingly, at his death, the healer declared that he would not transmit the *wereku* spirits; rather, he would send them back to the bush to await someone who passed by and pleased them. Ordinarily though, a spirit possessor will bequeath the spirit to a brother or sister's daughter. Spirits are never inherited in a direct line, e.g., mother to daughter. The most common procedure is that following the death of a person with spirits, family gather, together with cult leaders and musicians of the group in which the deceased had been initiated. For seven days, the family will dance, trudging round and round in a circle, accompanied by the appropriate instruments. From time to time, a dancer will appear to be possessed – her eyes will become fixed and she will become rigid and stay rigid even after the music stops. Several dancers may seem possessed during the inheritance dance period. As one observer put it:

> The spirits come, they try one person out, then another; the spirits tempt her, they come on her, leave, let her rest, return. They see how each one responds, who welcomes them best, and then they choose one.

After the ceremony, the cult leaders select the potential initiate but it may be years before the family proceeds with subsequent ceremonies to verify that the person has been chosen, due to the heavy expenses involved. If the ceremony is not held immediately following the death of a cult member, the need for its occurrence may be indicated by an episode or recurrence of illness afflicting a particular family member. In some instances, the occurrence of a person displaying certain symptoms such as vertigo, weakness, convulsions, or unusual behavior, may be suggestive of a spirit possession even if no relative can be remembered who left an uninherited spirit.

In the event that a ceremony is held to determine whether an illness is indicative of spirit possession, the symptoms should disappear after the afflicted person "falls," being surmounted by the spirit. In one case, an adolescent girl with a history of staring and behaving oddly, and thought to have a *sambani* spirit, was taken into the cult, and the spells ceased. On the other hand, a Fulbe woman was brought to a dance because she had been tearing off her waist cloth and running nude. A diviner who had been consulted as to the cause of this extreme behavior suggested she was bothered by a *sambani* spirit. At the dance, however, her spirit was very slow in coming and she refused to fall or show her eyes, the indicators of possession. Eventually people began to say that the woman wasn't possessed, she was "just crazy."

Dreams may also indicate that a spirit desires to be possessed. Thus Yaayi Yo, a cult leader, described her experience with the inheritance of a family *sambani* spirit.

> I got my spirit from my father's sister. This is normal. If you live a long life and die, you would leave your clothers to your brother's daughter. Then my father's sister came in a dream and showed me a white cloth and a sash to tie around my waist. I cried and went to Ya (former cult leader) to ask her what it meant. Ya told me to find the cloth, so I took cotton and made thread and had the cloth of the dream made. Then I danced in that cloth [and the spirits came.]

5.14. HEALING AND SAMBANI

The significance of spirit possession for the study of midwifery derives from the implications of the overlap between matrones and cult members, and more largely, the imputation of "power" to cult members. *Sambani* members, especially, are alleged to have special abilities and skills, ranging from divination to knowledge of words and substances. Because of the finding that individuals, particularly women, described by others as diviners or medicine people, were often also members of spirit cults, I was led to ask the question "are all *sambani* medicine people?" The answer to this question was categorically no. One diviner who is also a medicine person and a *sambani* leader explained the interrelationship by saying that certainly all *sambani* did not have medicine.

> Are children the same as adults? Within sambani, same are powerful and others are not. It's like European school. All want to succeed to become great but most don't. Only a few are powerful.

Within the cult, however, a person has potential access to other powerful individuals who may willing to share knowledge or take an apprentice. A cult member who has a matrone or who had an interest in pursuing this specialty might then apprentice herself to another more senior cult member who proved agreeable. Power, as defined by control of forces of good and evil, and capacity and knowledge to combat pathological agents, whether sent by spirits or men, is highly concentrated in the *sambani* membership. Thus cult membership provided contacts which would be tapped by prospective healers or healers seeking to augment their power.

What then, might be the direct contribution of spirit possession to a matrone's practice? *Bukakaaru*, because its effect is basically limited to the actual period of the possession state, would not provide a perpetual source of power to the matrone for strength in diagnosis and treatment, although being a cult member might be an attribute attracting clients. *Sambani*, on the other hand, might theoretically provide a means for a matrone to derive spiritual assistance. Some Bariba claim that those with spirits may be able to obtain help from them. First, no one, whether a person with spirits or not, can communicate directly with spirits or request assistance instantaneously. However, a *sambani* adept may be able to "see" the position of the child *in utero*, and to predict difficulties in a delivery. In general, healers who have spirits may also have the power to foresee the involvement of sorcery, or to advise on the treatment for illness via communications sent in dreams. Spirits may also send the knowledge of special healing words in the night. Thus indirectly, a woman who has *sambani* spirits may acquire knowledge and divination skills which would increase her capabilities as a matrone.

These increased capabilities are likely to promote the matrone to the status of healer (*tingi*) as opposed to simply "mother," or "one who does deliveries." The healer/technician distinction among matrones is primarily manifest in terms of degree of power and this is most often indicated by cult membership (especially *sambani*), which enables the matrone to draw on such assets as spirit contacts, clairvoyance, special words, in the practice of midwifery. One might, then, categorize birth assistants as the "attendant," who merely is present at a delivery and may perform such tasks as getting food or water for the parturient; the matrone, (*marusio*) who gives instructions and some remedies for complications of labor and delivery; and the matrone who is also a *tingi*, medicine person, who is most likely to have devoted more time to experimenting with medicines and learning special incantations and who is likely to be a spirit cult member.

Another correlation between midwifery and spirit possession of either the *sambani* or *bukakaaru* variety might be found in the character attributes which are a pre-requisite for both. The importance of strength of character for a spirit cult initiate is noted by numerous cult leaders and lay spectators. The conception of the spirits darting from individual to individual "testing" the various applicants and choosing the "best" is suggestive of the discrimination involved. The "best" or most suitable applicant requires such characteristics as courage, confidence, self-control and public presence. These qualities are necessary to carry the initiate through the ordeals of the testing rituals to verify the presence of the spirit, and the initiate is expected to suffer greatly before terminating the requirements. Such initiation ordeals include leaving the initiate immobilized on an anthill or termite mound – the truly possessed will not brush off the insects – or sending the initiates alone through the bush to find special objects such as sticks or cowrie shells which have been destined for them to find. Even the dancing required in the cult reunions necessitates the ability to shed the proverbial modesty of women and display oneself. Many women are reluctant to dance in ordinary festive dancing because they are "ashamed" or embarrased at being the object of attention but spirit cult members are obliged to dance while crowds gather to watch them. The speculation of one Bariba woman that those who have spirits on their heads lack "shame," then, seems to be an apt observation.

In the case of the matrone, the attributes of courage, self-confidence, presence, and authority are also desirable. The matrone may be obliged to make quick decisions, to give advice, to face death, pain, sorcery or witchcraft. The fear of "the things one might see" at a delivery inhibits many women from assisting, especially at a difficult birth where witchcraft is suspected. A matrone may risk blindness or illness from encounters with witch babies or affliction and even death from envy of others due to her position, or from anger due to her interventions. She also must lack shame in order to view another's nakedness.

In one instance, a midwife had her own praise-singer, who sang of her that "she is powerful, she will never need to 'eat shame" by her failure at a delivery." One observation related to this praising is that the praise-singer proceded to extemporaneously recite some obscene verses received with much hilarity by the midwife and her friends. Following the departure of the praise-singer, a Bariba woman commented that both praise-singers and women who possess spirits, such as the midwife in question, are without shame. The incident indicated the rarety of such praise-singing of a woman and the possible significance of spirit possession as a basis for respect. In this case both the praise-singing and the nature of the praises derive partly from the fact that this midwife is known for her powers as a spirit possession cult member, and not solely from her activities as "one who attends deliveries."

5.15. THE MATRONE PROTOTYPE

In the beginning of this chapter, it was suggested that a particular therapeutic option, such as a matrone or a nurse-midwife, is selected by a patient in order to accomplish a particular task; a client assumes that certain characteristics of the role occupant are requisite for the healer to be effective and competent. It seems likely that in the case of the matrone, she is perceived as competent because she possesses characteristics which are considered suitable to her role. This does not mean that every matrone will necessarily conform to an invariable set of rules, but that she will demonstrate attributes which fall within an acceptable range to the client. The review of social and career attributes of matrones has shown that there is a range of characteristics which are typical of a matrone and which render her acceptable in the perspective of her clientele.

In reviewing the characteristics of matrones, they were found to share the following attributes:

(1) For matrones, midwifery is a part-time speciality, one of a few avenues for women to increase their prestige. It does not provide primary income.

(2) Matrones are referred to as mother, not by a special title, but may be referred to descriptively as "one who does deliveries."

(3) Midwifery may be, but is not in all cases, a speciality subset of healers; the healer/technician distinction among matrones is primarily manifest in terms of degree of power, as indicated by knowledge of substances, words, and spirit cult membership. In this case, the midwife may be praised by praise-singers for her powers as a medicine person.

(4) Midwifery is not a hereditary occupation but is usually learned by apprenticeship from a mother or grandmother; spiritual call or assistance may also be a factor in selection and competence.

(5) Most matrones are animist.

(6) All are over 40 years of age; all except one was menopausal at her first unsupervised delivery.

(7) Only one had received formal education.

(8) All had been married at least once; approximately half were currently married; others were widows.

(9) Approximately 71% were wives of peasants (others were wives of chiefs or traders).

(10) All had at least two pregnancies and at least two living children.

(11) The majority specialized particularly in delivery assistance and child care.

(12) Slightly over 1/2 are Bariba commoners, 1/3 aristocrats.

One might predict then, that rural Bariba women expect that a competent matrone will resemble the prototype represented in the ensemble of these attributes. The significance of these characteristics becomes especially evident when one compares the typical government midwife to the matrone. The government midwife is likely to be a non-Bariba, with secondary school education; until very recently she was most likely to be a southerner transferred to work in the north, due to the small number of northern women who attended secondary school. She probably did not understand Bariba or Dendi (lingua franca of the region) and was in her early twenties. Most midwives, if married, were living without their families, often in a house alone or with a single relative, not in a typical family household. For the government midwife, midwifery is a full-time salaried job which places the midwife in the status group of civil service. This status affiliation dramatically separates the midwife from her client. Midwives, when married, are usually married to other civil servants, have no or few children, are of course literate, and learned medicine from books rather than apprenticeship. Many are Catholic or protestant, and if animist, do not participate in local rituals. Usually, the government midwife is addressed respectively by clients and neighbors as "*dokotoro*" (doctor, nurse); of course, being so young, most government midwives could not expect to be referred to as "mother" in any event.

The primary characteristics shared by matrones and government midwives is that both provide delivery assistance and treatment for early childhood ailments; however, the approach to treatment and to the client-practitioner relationship differs greatly. With regard to differences in responsibility and authority, for example, the nurse-midwife clearly pre-empts control of the situation. Contrastingly, the matrone may give advice and suggestions but her tone and actions are rarely ones of dominance; rather, she is in the role of supportive personnel – certainly possessed of esoteric knowledge, but not a controlling character. She speaks the same language as her patients, probably resembles their mothers or grandmothers, and shares the same sort of educational background, class background, household organization and marital status as her clientele and has a respectable reproductive history. Compared with the nurse-midwife, the matrone is notably more homophilous with her prospective patients. The nurse-midwife is most likely to give orders in French, thereby accentuating the social and cognitive distance between herself and her patients (manifest in her title of "*dokotoro*"); she may speak harshly and loudly, criticize the patient for not complying with instructions, being a "peasant," or for not "pushing" energetically enough. In general, she emphasizes the differences between herself as an educated, salaried, government employee, possibly a southerner – and her northern, uneducated, non-French-speaking clientele. Observation of the behavior of the nurse-midwife in the Kouande maternity clinic clearly indicated a difference between the nurse-midwife's treatment of southern women, usually wives of civil servants (who spoke French), her treatment of wealthy women, whether wives of civil servants or traders, and her treatment of local women who were wives of cultivators or small shopkeepers or traders. Rural women who had delivered in clinics often commented negatively both on the treatment they received, the attitude of the midwife, and on various attributes such as her age, ethnicity, marital status and also referred to her with the tone of fear and subdued demeanor with which most peasants react to government officials.

Finally, a note seems pertinent on cross-cultural studies of midwifery. In most societies, parturient women are assisted by birth attendants of varying degrees of specialization. According to Ford (1945), elderly women were found to assist at birth in 58 cultures of the 64 surveyed. In general, ethnographic data on status characteristics of midwives suggest that world-wide, indigenous midwives tend to be female, past middle-age, have been married, have had children, and learned by apprenticeship and/or divine calling (Ekanem et al. 1975; Cosminsky 1976). The Bariba, then, are unusual in their emphasis on the solitary delivery but the matrone prototype corresponds to that described for indigenous midwives in a variety of cultures.

CHAPTER 6

THE MEANING OF EFFICACY IN RELATION TO OBSTETRICAL CARE PREFERENCES

In preceding chapters, the argument was set forth that decisions regarding obstetrical assistance are influenced by cultural expectations, including generally shared concepts regarding the reproductive processes. Correspondingly, Bariba expectations regarding appropriate sociological and career attributes of matrones have implications for women's selection of a birth assistant. A further issue in the consideration of cultural expectation is the cultural meaning of "efficacy." This chapter will focus on the Bariba definition of birth as an event, on the ideal behavior for pregnant and delivering women, and on the implications of these expectations for the type of intervention which is likely to be considered necessary at birth based on the Bariba definition of effective and appropriate obstetrical therapy.

In order to interpret the pattern of utilization of birth assistance among the Bariba, one needs to begin with the assumption that in choosing among alternative medical services, choices are *ultimately* based upon the perception and meaning of the services to the client (Riley and Sermsri, 1974:52); the client also holds certain role expectations for the healer and acts according to the perceived meaning of the condition for which specialist intervention is sought. (This does not mean every matrone, as occupant of the status of matrone, will behave invariably according to a set role but that the clients can predict within a certain range her potential behavior.) Thus characteristics of the disorder, of the patient, of the healer, and of the service are all called into play as factors in decision-making with regard to obstetrical interventions.

In this chapter then, a primary hypothesis to be considered is that the selection of a particular medical service – in this case a maternity service – is largely derived from the diagnosis of the problem at hand and correspondingly that treatment of a disorder – in this instance obstetrical complications – is related to ideas of sickness causation.

Bariba expectations regarding the preferred type of intervention derive from the customary definition of the situation requiring intervention, in this case, childbirth. In general, the data suggest that:

(1) Bariba do not define pregnancy and normal delivery as a disease in the same sense of "an undesirable deviation in the way a person functions" (Fabrega 1974:298);

(2) in the event of a normal birth, the assistance of a specialist is not necessary;

(3) in the event of complications, birth becomes a life-threatening crisis requiring a specialist's intervention.

According to the Bariba, every woman should learn how to behave while pregnant; she should also learn simple medicines to ensure a safe, quick and easy delivery, and ideally, she should deliver alone. An unexpected finding was that according to ideal behavior, the woman should deliver unassisted. Contrastingly, a survey of the literature on midwives and reproduction suggests that in most societies a woman is assisted at the time of a delivery. Given that the Bariba norm is for a woman to deliver alone, should circumstances arise which lead her to seek help, her choice is made more dramatic by its variance from the ideal and the significance of the role of the assistant is emphasized. According to the ideal, however, even a primipara is expected to try to deliver without assistance. Information on primiparas is scant because of the difficulties encountered in interviewing them due to their reluctance to discuss reproduction. In the sample interviewed, about 40% of 120 women delivered their last child without any other person present until the baby delivered.[22] At that point, the woman called someone to cut the cord, or someone heard the baby crying and came for that purpose. Approximately 14% of the primiparas who responded delivered alone, compared to 43% of the multiparas.

Theoretically, all women are prepared to deal with a normal delivery. Pregnancy is not considered a disease, but rather a condition. One never hears "*u barɔ*" (she is sick) referring to a woman being pregnant. When a woman is said to be "sick" during her pregnancy, the meaning is likely to be similar to what is referred to in western medicine by the term "coincidental illnesses of pregnancy" (cf. Pritchard and Macdonald, Williams Obstetrics 1973:x). Those illnesses which are termed "illnesses of pregnancy" such as toxemia may or may not be considered to be associated with pregnancy by the Bariba, but if the statement "she is sick" is made, it is intended to indicate the occurrence of a complaint either separate from or additional to pregnancy. Thus, in response to the question "what sickness does she have?", the reply might be "she has abcess disease," "she has hernia," "she has stiff neck disease." One instance where a Bariba woman had a complaint which was considered to be associated with pregnancy was the case of Safura, a woman who experienced severe vomiting for the first five months of her pregnancy. In reference to Safura, people said "she has vomiting sickness" (because of, or with, her pregnancy) but not "she is sick." Others, however, doubted that the two were associated because the vomiting was so severe that it seemed to warrant being considered a sickness in its own right, rather than being considered the milder vomiting of early pregnancy.

A woman's knowledge of pregnancy is acquired not from healers who specialize in treating sickness but from more experienced women. A young married woman is informed by her aunts and grandmothers of cautions such as food taboos (large lizards are said to cause miscarriage, for example) and prohibited behavior such as walking outside at night when spirits are abroad which might harm the baby. A pregnant woman is likely to be told that she should work as hard as possible during her pregnancy so that at the hour of her delivery, her blood will not be thick and slow and inhiibit her labor. If she feels contractions, she should ignore them, and keep working; her family should also pretend not to notice. If she truly cannot work anymore, the woman chooses an empty room in which to rest but she is urged to walk around as much as possible. If she feels the urge to push, she should kneel, sitting on her heels. She should on no account touch or rub her back or stomach for fear of hurting the baby and she has undoubtedly been told since childhood that a woman who fusses or cries in childbirth dishonors her family and is lower than an ant. It is said that if a woman in labor wishes aloud that she had never become pregnant, she will henceforth become sterile.

If a pregnant woman is expected to be competent to deal with a normal birth, under what conditions did the 60% of the sample deliver who were assisted at their last delivery? The typical reasons given by Bariba for calling a matrone are:

(1) the woman is fearful;
(2) the woman has experienced difficult deliveries in the past;
(3) the delivery is in progress and is considered problematic.

In the latter two instances, the family and the delivering woman initially decide that the birth cannot be considered "normal." A matrone may then be called. The matrone's role thereafter is to study the symptoms and signs, define the situation, try to remedy any complications and assist the birth to progress.

A birth always has the potential for being abnormal, in spite of the fact that in the absence of complications, the intervention of a matrone is not required. A brief consideration of some Bariba sayings and counsel during pregnancy indicates the precarious state in which the pregnant woman is believed to dwell. Pregnant women are told that it is inappropriate to wear one's best jewelry and clothing while pregnant because of the imminence of death. A proverb states that "a pregnant woman is a dying person" (*guragi gɔri wa*) and another saying depicts the ancestors in the act of digging the woman's grave throughout her pregnancy. If she survives the delivery, they begin to shovel the sand back in and forty days after the delivery, the grave will finally be closed without her. In a conversation with a pregnant woman in her early 20's, the woman described herself as not in a position to argue over an issue, because, as she said, "do I know if the hour of my death is approaching?" Pregnancy, then, is a liminal state where the woman hovers between life and death and birth might well be defined as a normal but dangerous process, in which the risk of death is always present.

Contrastingly, in western medicine, birth is considered a "normal" physiological process but except under rare conditions, a delivery is a medical procedure. (Williams Obstetrics, for example, refers to a section on the "management of normal pregnancy and labor," and to a subsequent section on the abnormalities of labor, the puerperium, and so forth Pritchards and Macdonald 1976: Contents.) Thus, it is generally assumed that medical intervention is required at a delivery, whether or not complications occur. Frequently, pregnant women are classified by western physicians as low-risk or high-risk patients, but both require supervision, although different precautions would be taken for high-risk women depending on the problem involved.

To the Bariba, the delivery which most legitimately requires intervention is a "high-risk" delivery. This category most often includes the woman experiencing a problematic labor; the delivery is then termed "not good," meaning "not normal." Several fears are encompassed within the parameters of a delivery which does not follow the expected process. One apprehension is for the life of the mother, while a lesser fear is for the life of the child. The relative weight of each of these concerns is evident in the salutations appropriate at birth. If the child and the placenta are safely delivered and the mother is well, those present cry "*ka baraka*" (a blessing). If the baby is delivered safely but the placenta is retained, "*baraka*" is not heard, nor is it appropriate in the event the baby lives but the mother lives and the baby dies, one may still appropriately say "*baraka*" because the mother remains to carry the potential of delivering another child in the future.

The primary indicator of a delivery which is "not good" or "not normal" is that the child is born with the mark of the supernatural, in other words, the child is presumed to be a witch. Due to this possibility, those awaiting a birth always harbor an underlying anxiety that the child may present itself as a witch baby, (*bii yondo*) capable of killing its mother during delivery or of growing up to provoke havoc among patrilineal relations. An important function for the matrone, then, is to observe the delivery process and verify that labor is proceeding predictably; in other words, nothing unexpected or visibly abnormal is occurring which would lead one to await or fear a witch child. The matrone tries to prevent the death of the mother in case a witch child is attacking her; or she may call for the appropriate specialist in the event that a witch child is born. A matrone must have sufficient courage to deal with such catastrophic possibilities and enough discretion to never speak of what she has seen, even to the woman's husband, if this should be required.

The significance to the Bariba of detecting a witch child can be appreciated by the realization that witches represent one of the major causes of misfortune, together with poisoners, God, and malevolent spirits of the bush. An adult cannot become a witch; rather, a person is born with the power of witchcraft. Thus a Bariba elder, a former land chief of Pehunko respected for his knowledge of good and evil, explained that birth is the moment when a witch arrives on earth and must be apprehended. According to Bariba informants, the signs indicating a witch child are:

(1) a breech birth;
(2) child which slides on its stomach at birth;
(3) child born with teeth;
(4) child born with extreme birth defects;
(5) child born at 8 months (lunar months);
(6) or later on, a child whose teeth come in first in the upper gums.

These characteristics which signify abnormality to the Bariba are also considered abnormal in western obstetrics in the sense of being statistically less probable to occur. Thus 96% of births are predicted to be vertex presentations and less than 4% predicted to be breech births. Approximately 10% of deliveries are likely to terminate in a presentation where the baby might slide on its stomach, and very few babies are born with teeth.

One cannot assume that these statistics pertain without modification to developing countries or to the Bariba – for example, breech births increase with parity so that one might expect a higher percentage of breech births among Bariba than in Western Europe. However, breech births and presentations where baby slides on its stomach are nonetheless much less likely to occur than are vertex presentations or presentations where the baby slides on its back at delivery.

It seems then, that Bariba have a biomedically accurate perception of what constitutes the probable course of a delivery and the most frequently occurring types of presentations; births which deviate from this norm are then defined as abnormal and indicative of witchcraft.

Customarily, a child born with any of the above characteristics was killed shortly after birth.[23] The matrone, after verifying the situation, would call the funeral official (*gossiko*) or a male healer armed with protective medicines to administer poison to the child or to advise the mother not to feed the child but rather, to leave it to die. Of course it is difficult to quantify the number of such children born and/or not allowed to live. During a one and a half year period I learned of five such cases.

A witch baby may cause harm although it is never delivered as a live fetus. Such witch babies are thought responsible for grave complications of labor, particularly obstructed labor. Thus in one case, a woman died in labor before delivering the child. This form of death is perhaps the most dreaded, certainly by women, and in order to prevent its recurrence among other women, special ceremonies are prescribed. In this instance, when the woman died, after several matrones had tried futilely to save her, an old man was called to remove the child from her uterus prior to burial. This operation is required because two bodies should not be buried in one grave. When the child was removed, it is alleged, it was alive, very large, had all its teeth, and was smiling. Whenever this case is recounted in discussions on the risks of birth, people remark "now that was a child which killed its mother." While the old man was preparing the burials, all the women of the village who were pregnant or carrying babies on their backs fled into the bush, wailing, after throwing out all cooked food, emptying water jars, and extinguishing fires. They would not return until the gravediggers finished filling in the graves, at which time ordinary household activities could commence anew. One might wonder by what means, if witch babies are destroyed at birth, do any adult witches remain. The answer seems to lie in the fact that it is debatable whether a child defined as a witch is actually killed; first, if a woman delivers alone, and, for example, the child slides on its stomach, she might theoretically decide to move it into another position before someone arrived to cut the cord. Bariba questioned on this subject agreed that a woman who could bear the risks and keep a secret forever in her heart might do such a thing. It is not impossible that a matrone might also connive in such a fashion. Some breech births, depending on the point of view of the specialists whose opinion is sought, might be defined as acceptable. In these and similar ways, a dangerous child might slip through the screening mechanisms and live to grow up and cause harm.

The significance of witch children in affecting decisions regarding obstetrical assistance should not be under-estimated. Delivering alone provides a woman and her family with flexibility of options – the woman who delivers without assistance may, as described above, try to alter the situation; a matrone present at an "abnormal" birth may assist the mother by trying to protect her from the witch child. If a witch child is delivered, the matrone may then call another specialist to deal with the situation (kill the child, decide to give it away to the Fulbe or the *gossiko* or to let it die). In no event will the matrone divulge the truth outside those immediately involved. Relatives and neighbors might be told that the woman had delivered a stillborn child. Thus the options fall in both directions: flexibility to keep or destroy the child.

On the other hand, if a woman delivers at a maternity clinic, her options seem more limited. First, the delivery is more public than a home delivery. However, usually the woman delivers in a room with only the clinic personnel present; the relative or friend who accompanied her is not allowed in the room. Women often asserted that the government midwife, especially when she is a member of a different ethnic group, is not aware of the importance of identifying a dangerous child. Because the mother is obliged to deliver lying down, rather than in the Bariba style of kneeling, she herself cannot determine in what position the child is delivered, in order to determine if it is a breech birth or other presentation, if she delivered a healthy child, it would be difficult to poison it or to not feed it while at the maternity clinic. Although theoretically it is possible to do so, most people today are concerned with the likelihood of being reported to the *gendarmes* (police) or army, and sanctioned.

The effect of this restriction of options is to cause some women to hesitate before delivering at the maternity clinic. This hesitation was articulated by women in the district of Kerou, where several young women were trained to be auxiliary midwives to do home deliveries by Catholic nuns of nursing order. One young trained auxiliary said that women were reluctant to call her to assist them at deliveries because they feared it was "like going to a maternity clinic." However, they woman continued, she had tried to reassure them that what she saw at a delivery would never be divulged, and some seemed to believe and accept her. After lengthy discussion, it became clear that what the village women feared was (a) that she would force them to lie down to deliver, which is disliked for a variety of reasons, among them the restriction of visibility of the child's position at delivery, and (b) that she would either spread the news of an abnormal birth or report it to the authorities.

To some Bariba, the implications of maternity deliveries and the interference of government authorities are awesome. The former Land Chief of Pehunko, for example, bemoaned the fact that with all the witch children alive and running around today, especially in urban areas, there are probably 20 to 30 deaths a month provoked by these children. One might, for example, be walking around the market place, eating, and a witch child might become jealous and cause a misfortune.

To recapitulate, then, many Bariba women prefer an indigenous matrone if they experience obstetrical complications, because of expectations regarding the type of intervention likely to be necessary at birth. These expectations derive from the definition of birth as a normal but dangerous state, which signifies the omnipresent potential for the triumph of abnormality, evil and disorder. Correspondingly, the function of the competent matrone is to provide effective therapy as defined by the ability to diagnose and deal with abnormal births and refer the patient when the matrone's level of competence is surpassed.

The concept of effective therapy among the Bariba is not necessarily congruent with that of western medicine, although it is possible that some Bariba cures produce physiological changes which would also be considered "cures" in biomedicine. More pertinent than physiological effects of curing is the distinction remarked by Young between hopes and expectations. A cure *sometimes* fulfills the hope of the sick person for restoration to better health but an "established cure is always able to work in the sense that it meets the expectations of the sick person and his kin and that it produces certain results in a predictable way" (Young 1976:7). People utilize their medical practices, he states, "because the practices are empirically effective . . . this is not the same thing as saying that (1) the practices are effective from the standpoint of Western medical notions or that (2) the practices always bring the results (e.g., remissions of symptoms) for which the people themselves hope" (7).

Bariba delivery beliefs and practices illustrate Young's contention that healing may be perceived as efficacious in that a diagnosis or prognosis is verified rather than an expected physiological change produced, or a biomedically correct explanation of an even provided. Thus a healer may be characterized as knowledgeable because in retrospect a prediction made by that healer seems accurate. A clear illustration of an instance in which the prediction is correct but the explanation is not biomedically accurate involves one type of which baby. Mention was made previously of the belief that a baby which slides on its stomach as it is expelled is a baby with powers of witchcraft. Some matrones warn pregnant or delivering women that a woman who grimaces and fusses in labor will *cause* the baby to slide on its stomach. The effect of this prediction is that in some cases, a mother is held to be responsible for delivering a witch baby.

A biomedical interpretation of this sequence might be that the woman delivered a child in an unreduced occipito-posterior presentation or in a face presentation. That is, the baby would be delivered with its face towards the mother's stomach and as the baby rotates so that its shoulders can be delivered, its body will continue to turn with the force of the rotation. If, as is customary, no one catches the baby, it will slide along the floor on its stomach. Moreover, in the unreduced occipito-posterior and face presentations, labor may be prolonged (Myles 1971:341). The mother may complain of exhaustion, backache, and other discomforts. The greater possibility of prolonged and uncomfortable labor in such presentations suggests a greater likelihood of grimacing and other expressions of discomfort by the mother during labor. In sum, *because* of the type of presentation, the woman grimaced. This explanatory statement of the relationship is the inverse of the Bariba prediction that if a woman grimaces, she will *cause* a baby to slide on its stomach.

In addition, it is interesting to note that in the event of a birth where the baby fell on its stomach and witchcraft was suspected, the baby may carry marks from the delivery which support this diagnosis. Thus an English midwifery text, in a discussion on nursing the newborn delivered in a face presentation, states that "the face is congested and bruised, the eyelids and lips oedematous . . . if, the blue discoloration and the disfiguring oedema are excessive, the mother should not see her baby until they have subsided" (Myles 1971: 381). Such swelling and disfigurement such as moulding of the head would tend to substantiate preliminary impressions that a newborn was a dangerous child.

In general, in comparing the roles of the matrone and the government midwife, one finds overlap in the provision of a technical function. Both specialists work towards the same outcome – delivery of the child. However government midwives interpret the implications of birth more narrowly than do the matrones and many of their clients. In the Bariba case, then, indigenous midwifery encompasses a complex of beliefs and practices not paralleled by the profession of nurse-midwifery as practiced in a clinic setting. The role of nurse-midwife is lacking in dimensions in comparison with the comprehensive technical, ritual and social functions of the matrone. From the perspective of clients, the alternative of nurse-midwifery for birth assistance would not be selected because it could not be expected to solve the problem as defined by most Bariba.

Increasingly, research on patient-practitioner relationships has demonstrated that decisions to select particular therapeutic options, and compliance with therapeutic regimes are influenced by the extent to which patients and practitioners share fundamental assumptions regarding clinical reality. This general conclusion has been thoroughly illustrated by Kleinman (1978a, b); and for Africa, the review of health care systems by Good et al. has provided additional evidence that "cultural empathy and value consonance between patient and healer" are of primary significance to therapeutic efficacy (Good et al. 1979: 143).[24]

Documentation for this contention from the cross-cultural study of midwifery is thus far slim, but several substantiating examples exist. Jordan, for instance, argues that

> A society's way of conceptualizing birth constitutes the single most powerful indicator of the general shape of its birthing system . . . This locally shared view of childbirth guarantees that, by and large, participants have similar views regarding the course and management of birth (Jordan 1978:34).

Her comparison of birth practices in the United States, Yucatan, Holland, and Sweden relates "locally shared views of childbirth" to prevailing obstetrical procedures in those societies.

Similarly, Dorothea Sich discusses obstetrics in rural Korea, where a rural health care project offered special emphasis on maternity care, including free midwife attendence. Nonetheless, project evaluation indicated that midwife attendance at birth had not risen substantially. The author suggests that "offered services in maternity care are not acceptable to the cultural conditions under which the recipients live" (Sich 1979:1). These conditions include the expectation that childbearing is a family responsibility, rather than that of the individual woman.

The pregnant woman is not considered to be sick, and families disapprove of interference from "outside;" families also protest some practices prevalent in cosmopolitan obstetrics such as the lithotomy position. Moreover, admiration is expressed for women who give birth alone. In general, the author concludes that childbearing is a kind of initiation rite (4). Because cosmopolitan medicine ignores or belittles the tenets of the indigenous obstetrical system, parturients and their families hesitate to utilize the offered services, even when midwife attendance was free of charge.

A further example where parturients and meedical practitioners manifest widely divergent views regarding efficacious maternity care is provided by Pillsbury (1978), who describes Chinese women in Taiwan who categorically refused to enter an air-conditioned delivery room or allow air-conditioning in a maternity ward because of the traditional Chinese practice of "doing the month." According to this tradition, for one month post-partum, women should be confined to home, and observe behaviors intended to remedy pregnancy-induced hot-cold imbalance (Pillsbury 1978:11). In the United States, adherence to the practice of "doing the month" leads some Chinese-American women hospitalized for maternity care to reject certain foods and procedures recommended by western medical personnel. Pillsbury concludes that the persistence of these post-partum practices both in Taiwan and in the People's Republic of China indicates that new techniques must be integrated with indigenous traditions in order to provide health services which are respectful of indigenous beliefs and practices retaining widespread significance for patients.

Morsy, describing childbirth in an Egyptian village, offers an additional case which substantiates the contention that divergent models of clinical reality affect selection of obstetrical care options (in press). Morsy notes that rural women prefer to deliver at home with a midwife except in the event of a difficult birth (21). Informants criticized health service physicians for being mean and mocking peasants and for behaving inappropriately to women in labor (see also Frankel 1977 for an extended case study of American women whose views regarding childbearing differ greatly from the "medical model").

Finally, it is useful to refer to a recent publication from the Johns Hopkins University Population Information Program on "Traditional Midwives and Family Planning (May, 1980). In summary, the report states:

> The traditional health sector, both urban and rural, consists of a great variety of indigenous practitioners, including traditional midwives, who live close to their clients, dispense herbs, potions, massage and other familiar remedies on request and take time to provide conventional wisdom and personal services for people who speak the same language, both literally and figuratively, and often come from the same background. For most villagers and many city dwellers in developing countries, going to a traditional practitioner is more comfortable, more convenient, and usually less expensive than going to a physician or hospital" (J-441).

The Bariba example, then, is not merely an isolated case where obscure witchcraft beliefs deter women from utilizing cosmopolitan maternity services. Rather, the Bariba exemplify a situation where the definition of the "event" directs patients to a particular treatment option. Decisions concerning obstetrical care are influenced by beliefs regarding the reproductive processes; ideal behavior for pregnant women; and assumptions about the causation of misfortune. Matrones and pregnant women share a model of clinical reality in which the threat of withcraft at delivery is an integral element.

In discussing the cultural construction of clinical reality, Kleinman et al. have stated that "Through diagnostic activities and labeling, health care providers negotiate with patients medical 'realities' that become the object of medical attention and therapeutics" (Kleinman et al. 1978a:254). The definition of the event and associated concepts regarding diagnosis and treatment comprise critical elements of such medical realities. A consideration of Bariba obstetrics suggests that the degree to which these models of clinical reality are shared by patients and practitioners strongly influences client's choices of practitioners and health services.

CHAPTER 7

BIRTH ASSISTANCE IN THE RURAL AREA: PATTERNS OF DELIVERY ASSISTANCE

According to the Bariba ideal, a pregnant woman during her first pregnancy will be tutored by relatives and friends in appropriate behavior and interdictions. During subsequent pregnancies, she is expected to be self-sufficient and not to need counsel except in the event of abnormalities. Additionally, the ideal woman delivers alone, calling for assistance to cut the cord after the delivery of the child. Even a primipara is expected to try to deliver alone.

The significant issue under consideration in this section is: do women actually conform to the ideal? For what purposes do women call for assistance? Do women request delivery assistance or only cord-cutting or baby-washing? What is the relationship of such assistants to the parturient? The actual pattern of selection of birth attendants will be examined. Subsequently, the second part of the chapter will entail a consideration of midwifery as a therapeutic system, and the implications of this for utilization of birth attendants. Structured interviews will be reviewed as will cases where delivery assistance was sought, with the intent of delving into the factors influencing women to (1) choose to have a birth attendant as opposed to a solitary delivery and (2) choose a matrone in preference to (or in conjunction with) national health personnel.

7.1. DELIVERY ASSISTANCE: PATTERNS OF SELECTION IN THE RURAL AREA

In order to determine the pattern of selection of birth attendants, 117 women were interviewed regarding (1) Person Present at Last Delivery; (2) Neighborhood of Last Birth Attendant; (3) Relationship Between Cord-Cutter and Parturient; (4) Neighborhood of Cord-Cutter; (5) Relationship of Baby Washer and Parturient; (6) Neighborhood of Baby Washer. These categories were selected following a pretest of the survey for women of reproductive age. A general question regarding the birth assistant present at the woman's most recent delivery elicited responses indicating (a) whether the woman delivered alone; (b) who cut the cord; (c) who washed the baby. In order to separate these responses and to differentiate type of birth assistance, women were interviewed regarding each of the above categories. Relationship between specialist and client and neighborhood of each were considered significant areas for questioning in order to trace possible kinship or residential bases for selecting a birth attendant.

The women interviewed reside in nine "neighborhoods" of the village of Pehunko. These neighborhoods are: Sinawararu, Gberasson, Borgou, Zongo, Pehunko Center, Banikani, Haske, Tance and Gbankerou. Although these neighborhoods are officially integrated in the village of Pehunko, residents sometimes identify themselves as residents of those neighborhoods, rather than as inhabitants of Pehunko. This identification with the neighborhoods was particularly evident with respect to Tance, Gbankerou and Sinawararu. Respondents to a questionnaire which requested information on place of birth, marriage, parents' origins, etc. often answered with the name of one of the above neighborhoods and not by indicating "Pehunko" as the response.

These three neighborhoods are spatially somewhat separate from Pehunko. Tance and Gbankerou are located approximately one kilometer beyond the entrance to Pehunko from the east while Sinawararu is located approximately the same distance beyond the western extent of the village. Gberasson is another village section often cited by residents as an identifying location; until fairly recently (probably within the past 15 years) Gbersson was a village "in the bush." It then displaced itself to join Pehunko "on the main road," apparently at government instigation. Many villages throughout Benin have migrated in this fashion in order to comply with government regulations developed to facilitate tax collection and nationalism.

The distribution of respondents in the sample of women interviewed regarding selection of birth attendants is not proportionate to the distribution of population in these neighborhoods, partly because of the lack of data on population size in the various sections and partly because of the necessity of using those respondents who agreed to participate in the survey, regardless of residence. It is, nonetheless, possible to distinguish some differences among neighborhoods which seem reasonable and in line with available data concerning these settlements. This will be discussed further below.

7.1.1. *Person Present at Last Delivery*

Of 117 cases reviewed, 38% delivered their last child alone, without any other person present during labor and delivery. The parturient then typically called for assistance in cutting the cord and/or supervising the delivery of the placenta. Of those 62% who were assisted, 25% were attended by either a "grandmother" or an "old lady," (often referred to as "my old lady" by the parturient). The majority of these old ladies were either paternal grandmothers or classificatory grandmothers or female relatives of the woman's husband. The next largest category of assistance was the male village nurse (22% of those cases attended by someone).[25]

Utilization of the nurse might be explained in terms of the preference for solitary deliveries except where complications arise. The cases where the nurse was called tended to be perceived as complicated and the nurse was usually sought after an "old lady" or a matrone had been called, except in the cases from Zongo neighborhood, to be discussed below. Following "nurse" in numerical importance was "mother." This category is particularly interesting because of the "ideal" avoidance between a biological mother and her child which prohibits the mother from assisting at her child's delivery due to "shame" (*sekuru*). In this sample, 14% of the birth attendants were "mothers"; it is possible, however, that some were not real mothers although an attempt was made to assure that the birth attendant was referred to as "*mero*" (biological mother) rather than "*yaayi*," (generic term for a person who stands in the position of mother to ego, e.g., mother's sisters, cousins and sometimes grandmother's generation as well). Two of the mothers in question were Yoruba, and would not be subject to the avoidance ideal, but with regard to the others, sufficient data are unfortunately not available to interpret the meaning of their presence.

The final major category of birth attendant is "mother-in-law" (11%). In addition, persons in a variety of other relationships to the parturient were sometimes present to assist her; these include older sister (6%); mother's sister (4%); co-wife (4%); patrilateral parallel cousin (1%); uncle's wife (1% – exact link unspecified); husband's sister (1%); father's wife (1%) and brother's wife (1%). The variety of persons present in a household to assist at a delivery reflects the heterogeneity of household composition; the apparent preference for an old lady to attend a delivery if assistance was sought seems likely to be related to the beliefs that elderly people are more competent to deal with situations requiring healing skills. The elderly are, in addition, more knowledgeable in coping with supernatural forces which may manifest themselves at a delivery. The particular relationship between the elderly birth attendent and the parturient may depend on whether the parturient remains in her husband's household or returns to the household where she grew up. In her husband's household, she is likely to be living with his mother, father, possibly his brothers and their spouses, and an assortment of other relatives of varying degrees of distance. The birth attendant, if any, will usually be drawn from these readily accessible individuals.

In only five cases, the birth attendant was specified as a matrone (all five were in Zongo neighborhood where ethnic differences may have influenced the responses – see below). The fact that only five attendants were referred to as matrones is not necessarily significant in reflecting either the occurrence of complications or choice of a specialist to deal with complications. Rather, it may reflect the great reluctance to cite the name of a matrone or implicate a matrone in a treatment process in an interview with an European. Although I have confidence that the relationships described in answer to the question "who assisted you at your last delivery?" are accurate, I suspect that respondents did not fully indicate which "old ladies" were matrones, and in which cases a matrone attended the delivery before the nurse was called. The number of matrone-assisted deliveries, then, is probably under-reported.

In considering differences in patterns of utilization among neighborhoods, one finds two notable distinctions. One is that in the neighborhood of Zongo, only two of 15 respondents (16%) delivered without assistance and 5/15 women claimed that a matrone attended their delivery. This contrasts greatly with the general proportion (38%) of women who delivered without assistance. An explanation for this difference is probably the number of Djerma, Hausa, and Niger Fulbe women living in that neighborhood, who rely more on a birth attendant and idealize less the solitary delivery than do Bariba women. The Bariba matrone who serves the Zongo area articulated this interpretation of the situation, saying that the women of her neighborhood were "less courageous" than Bariba women and didn't like to deliver alone.

A second distinction evident in a neighborhood is the selection of mothers-in-law and older sisters as birth attendants in most cases where a woman sought assistance in Sinawararu. I cannot explain this preference at this point. Sinawararu also had the largest number of women who delivered alone (14/26). A presentation of the neighborhood pattern is shown in Table 7.

TABLE 7
Birth attendants by neighborhood (major categories).

Neighborhood	Not assisted	Mother in-law	Old lady	Older sister	Mother	Nurse	Total
Sinawararu	14	4	3	4	0	0	25
Gberasson	5	0	2	0	0	0	7
Borgou	12	0	5	0	2	4	23
Zongo	2	0	5	0	0	5	12
Pehunko Center	2	2	0	0	0	4	8
Tance	0	0	0	0	2	1	3
Haske	9	0	0	0	4	2	15
Banikani	0	1	0	0	0	0	1
Gbankerou	2	0	8*	0	0	0	10
Total	46	7	23	4	8	16	104

*Relative of husband of parturient.

Approximately 77% of the birth attendants lived in the same household as the parturient, 19% resided in the same neighborhood but not in the same household, and in only one case was the person who assisted at the delivery from a different neighborhood (a mother from Tance came to her daughter's delivery in Haske, about 3/4 mile walk).

7.1.2. *Clients and Cord-Cutters*

In 19% of 116 cases of deliveries for which the information exists, the cord was cut by the village nurse. In the remaining 81% of the cases, the primary figures who cut the cord were in 11% of the cases an "old lady," (exact relationship unknown except in three cases where she was the parturient's father's mother); in another 11% of the cases, the husband's mother cut the cord; and in 13% of the cases, the cord-cutter was the mother of the parturient. Of the remainder, 6% were cut by a sister, 3% by a co-wife, 3% by a neighbor, 3% by a father's sister, 1% by a father's brother's wife, 1% by a father's father, and 1% by a husband's sister. In addition, four elderly women who are known as specialists (three at least are matrones but one claimed she had no medicines and only cut cords and washed babies) were called in 25% of the cases. These women practice primarily within the neighborhood where they live. Thus one finds matrones practicing as is shown in Table 8 (based on reports by women of reproductive age regarding assistance at their most recent delivery).

TABLE 8
Matrones as cord-cutters by neighborhood

Neighborhood	Matrones			
	Adama	Ganigi	Yon Seko	Bore
Haske	2	0	0	0
Borgou	9	0	0	0
Zongo	0	6	0	1
Gbankerou	0	0	9	0
Pehunko Center	0	0	0	1
Gberasson	0	1	0	0

Haske and Borgou are adjoining neighborhoods and Adama tends to serve the overlapping area radiating around her concession. In one case, Adama was the mother-in-law of the parturient. Ganigi practices mainly in Zongo, the foreigner's neighborhood. The Gberasson case involved a woman who lived directly across the main road from Zongo at the outskirts of the Gberasson area. In two cases, Ganigi was related to the parturient or linked to the family; as the mother's sister to one parturient and via her husband (a Hausa) to another parturient's husband. Yon Seko works predominately in Gbankerou (although she is called to Tance, across the road, as well). Bore is the sole exception to the pattern; she lives at the juncture of Borgou and Haske, in the concession of the former chief of Pehunko, as first wife. In both cases where she cut the cord, she was the husband's father's wife. Bore is best known for healing and for spirit possession rather than for cord-cutting or baby-washing; in fact, she has never been known to wash babies, even in the rare instances where she cut the cord.

In sum, in 97 cases for which the information exists, 47% of the cord-cutters came from the same neighborhood as the parturient; 36% from the same household; 14% were uncertain responses; and 2% were from different neighborhoods. In comparison, of persons "present at last delivery," 77% were from the same household; 19% from the same neighborhood. The implication seems to be that outsiders tend to be called to cut the cord more frequently than to assist at a delivery, although one must also consider that those women who delivered alone are obviously not included in the sample with "person present at last delivery" but all had a cord-cutter. However, it is still interesting that in spite of the often-expressed statement that "any courageous person can cut the cord," the person present at the delivery apparently did not always do so. As the table below shows, some birth attendants did cut the cord, but in 25% of the cases, a specialist was called to perform this task. This division of labor may perhaps be related to the belief that a person who assists at a delivery and lingers to cut the cord and/or wash the baby may go blind.

TABLE 9
Birth attendants and cord-cutters by relationship to client

Birth attendants by relationship (major categories)			Cord-cutters by relationship (major categories)
no assistant	39%		–
husband's mother	11%		11%
"old lady"	25%	"unspecialized"	11%
		specialist	25%
older sister	6%		6%
mother	14%		13%
nurse	22%		19%

7.1.3. *The Baby-Washer*

As with cord-cutters, approximately 23% of the baby-washers were specialists, known for their skill at this practice. If one counts the well-known specialists and other neighbors not so widely renowned, the proportion rises to 32%.

TABLE 10
Baby-washer by relationship to client

Baby washer by relationship (major categories)	
specialist-neighbor	23%
"old lady" of house	18%
mother	14%
husband's mother	9%
neighbor (not renowned)	9%
unspecified	9%
misc. kin	17%

Comparing the geographical relationship of the clients and baby-washers, one sees that the majority of the washers were from the same neighborhood, but not from the same household.

TABLE 11
Neighborhood of client and baby-washer

	Same house	Same neighborhood	Diff. neigh.	?
#	22	81	1	13
%	19	69	1	11

A comparison of the residences of person assisting at last delivery, cord-cutters, and washers indicates a diminishing proportion of assistants from within the household – 77% from the same household in the case of person present; 36% in the case of the cord-cutter; and 19% of baby-washers residing in the same household as the client. The specialist baby-washers, Adama, Ganigi, Seko, Ya, and Manou practiced primarily within their own neighborhoods as was found to be true for cord-cutters.

TABLE 12
Baby-washers by neighborhood

	Baby-washer				
Neighborhood	Adama	Ganigi	Seko	Ya	Manou
Borgou	12	0	0	0	0
Pehunko Center	3	0	0	0	0
Haske	2	0	0	0	0
Gberasson	0	1	0	0	0
Zongo	0	6	0	1	0
Gbankerou	0	0	9	0	0

Although it was not possible to do a thorough comparative study of patterns of birth assistance by collecting data in another village, some available information on the village of Doh provides material for speculation. Doh is a primarily non-Muslim Bariba village, population approximately 800, located approximately 18 kilometers from Pehunko, off the main road. Because of the lack of national health infrastructure and its generally isolated location and slow communications flow, Doh provides a useful comparison for Pehunko, with its more heterogeneous population – Muslim, Bariba, commoner, aristocrat, migrants; national government presence – in considering the selection of birth assistances. Moreover, Doh provides a useful contrast to Pehunko because certain rituals such as one type of ceremony for a new baby, have not been performed in Pehunko for perhaps 20 years whereas Doh residents continue to observe the rituals. Thus the situation in Doh is suggestive of the pattern of birth practices in Pehunko prior to the growth in population, increase in migrants from various ethnic groups, increasing Islamization, etc.

Doh remains an isolated village, fairly remote from the variations introduced by the national government, due to the exceedingly poor road which is unusable for three months of the year, and which requires a determined effort to travel at any season. Doh, to this date, has no school or on-side nurse; children either live with relatives in other villages or travel six kilometers by foot daily to the nearest school. Doh residents have little interaction with Europeans; when I visited a circumciser to ask questions about female circumcision, she consulted a diviner after my departure in great concern over the meaning of my visit. There are few commercial goods for sale in Doh – no tomato paste or peanut oil – staples in Pehunko; sauce recipes are simple and "old-fashioned" to some Pehunko women who refer to a trip to Doh as "going to the bush." Health care is provided Doh residents periodically by the itinerant, endemic diseases nurse or in the event of an emergency or a person seeking immediate consultation, the usual procedure is for the individual in ill health to travel or be brought to Pehunko.

Interestingly, no woman from Doh is recorded as having delivered in either the Pehunko dispensary or the Kouande district maternity clinic in any existing records. Currently, Doh is served by two elderly matrones; for this study, three were interviewed, including the two still practicing and one who is blind and no longer assists at deliveries. Information on Doh was acquired primarily from these midwives, and from selected women with whom I stayed during trips to Doh, Doh residents in Pehunko and miscellaneous other Doh residents.

The village of Doh is composed of three sections, or neighborhoods. Each of these neighborhoods was principally served by one of the now elderly matrones; the two remaining in practice share the village since the retirement of their contemporary. Of these two, one is alleged to be the most powerful and the most charitable. The other (Gbira), wife of the former chief of Doh, is said to resent being called out at night and to generally be less helpful a person than her colleague, Yon Sika. Yon Sika, who was perhaps the most forthcoming of all the matrones interviewed, outlined the pattern of birth assistance in Doh as follows: first, a woman tries to deliver by herself for a day or perhaps two. Then she calls the matrone in her neighborhood and usually in a truly difficult case, Yon Sika will be called. She claims she has never lost a mother or had to evacuate a patient; in one case, she did send a cyclist for the nuns to drive in and transport a woman, but the woman delivered before they arrived. Until recently, when Yon Sika felt her skill was surpassed, she called a male healer, Dogi, now deceased. He in turn (according to Yon Sika and his niece) only lost one patient and that a very small woman whom he had already advised not to have another child. She died in obstructed labor.

Dogi is an example of a healer whose fame extended byond his immediate locale. It is this category of healer who may be called if a neighborhood matrone cannot deal with a complicated case. Similarly, a matrone from Soaodou is called to treat women in Fwabwereku (her mother's village) 12 kilometers away. Specialists in sterility are also known throughout the region. Dogi, the healer from Doh, was also known regionally but ordinarily, the village limits are not surpassed in seeking obstetrical care, except in instances of serious complications. One exception is the village of Gbeke, where two matrones died within a short period and in the event of difficult births, a matrone in Tokoro, three kilometers away, is requested to help.

In a large village such as Pehunko and even Doh, several matrones were found practicing concurrently, organized loosely by neighborhood, usually with an understood order of competence. In a small village, matrones claimed that is difficult for more than one matrone to practice, and an apprenticeship type of arrangement may be established, wherein one matrone follows another and the superior in status instructs the subordinate in what procedures to follow, sends her to collect herbs and so forth. Sometimes, if the superior is called to a delivery but is unable to attend, the subordinate will supervise the delivery alone. This apprenticeship relationship is not always a function of the size of the settlement. For example, in Soaodou (population 800) and Sayakrou (population 700–800), two matrones work more or less together in each village. In each case, one is known as the superior and the other as less powerful, but both have their own apprentices.

The subordinate matrone of the Sayakrou pair said that Sayakrou was "too small" to have two independent matrones so that one was obliged to "follow" the other. In actuality, however, size may not be the factor. The village of Doh, with more or less the same population, supports two independent matrones and had three in the past. If size is not the factor, how can this arrangement be explained? One possible explanation involves status characteristics of the matrones. In this case, the characteristic of membership in a spirit cult seems to be a common factor with explanatory value. In the instance of Doh, where the three matrones practiced independently, none of the three belonged to spirit cults. One was a commoner, and the other two were aristocrats but this distinction did not appear significant. In Soaodou, the superior midwife was also a renowned spirit cult member; she possessed a powerful instrument, a stick of polished wood carved and covered with cowrie shells, and named "*duro toko*," (old man). She used this stick in dancing at cult reunions and also in treating complications of labor. Her colleague is also a cult member but is a much younger woman, of lesser renown. This younger woman is sometimes called for deliveries alone, but often the elder is called first. Even if the younger is called first, it is nonetheless understood that she is less qualified. In Sayakrou, the two matrones always work together unless the superior requests that the subordinate go alone to a delivery. Of these two matrones, the superior is a spirit cult member but the subordinate is not. It is interesting to note that in these and other cases of two matrones working together (though it should be emphasized that the typical procedure is for one healer to work alone and if no success occurs, another will arrive and the first one leave), it may happen that the more powerful matrone is called first, in contrast to the general pattern described earlier where the less powerful assistant is approached first and her skills exhausted prior to escalation to a more powerful healer.

The data from Pehunko, then, suggest that approximately 40% of the women interviewed delivered their most recent child alone and subsequently called for assistance in cutting the cord and sometimes for delivery of the placenta. Of these women who were assisted, 15% were attended by an elderly female relative and other attendants included "mothers," sisters, co-wives, and a variety of other female relatives. Approximately 77% of birth assistants came from the same household as the parturient and 19% who were not from the household came from the same neighborhood. Contrastingly, only 36% of cord-cutters came from the same household. Similarly, the majority of baby-washers came from the same neighborhood but not from the same household.

Although reproductive histories were not taken in Doh, the pattern of birth assistants as indicated by matrones and other informants provides supplementary evidence for the pattern apparent in Pehunko.

In sum, the example of the pattern in Doh provides supplementary evidence of the pattern apparent in Pehunko; brief examples from other villages such as Sayakrou and Soaodou also are suggestive in explaining the relationships of matrones to one another. The data suggest that: a woman attempts delivering without assistance. If she delivers successfully, she calls for help with the cord. If she needs help with the placenta or for complications of labor, first she is likely to call a family member, and next a specialist from the neighborhood. If the neighbor fails, a more powerful person from any neighborhood will be sought. This hierarchy of ascending power was explained by one informant who said that you don't escalate until you need to; you don't go to the provincial hospital if the local nurse can care for you and you don't call a powerful healer to deal with a simple problem.

7.2. MIDWIFERY AS A THERAPEUTIC SYSTEM

The existing literature on midwifery does not generally indicate clearly whether midwifery techniques and practices are idiosyncratic, varying from midwife to midwife, or a therapeutic system common to midwives practicing within a given culture. Although cross-cultural studies of midwifery refer to "Mayan" midwives or "Kentucky" midwives, implying that midwifery represents a culturally specific form of therapy, this issue is not directly addressed. This section, then, will consider the proposition that Bariba midwifery is a therapeutic system comprising shared beliefs, values, practices and techniques.

Support for the proposition that midwifery is a therapeutic system will be presented first from a consideration of detailed interviews with 19 matrones and, in addition, descriptions of matrones engaged in assisting at deliveries. Subsequently, cases demonstrating client-practitioner encounters will be presented. These cases are intended to further substantiate the hypothesis that Bariba midwifery is a therapeutic system. The discussion of interviews with matrones and case reports are in general intended to provide a basis for discussing the suggestion that client choice of birth assistance is affected by assumptions shared with matrones regarding the practice of midwifery.

7.3. STRUCTURED INTERVIEWS WITH MATRONES

The following consideration of some midwifery concepts, techniques and practices is based on both structured interviews and informal discussions held with 19 matrones, residing in 6 Bariba villages. These women were interviewed regarding experiences with delivering women, and problems encountered in pregnancy, labor, and the post-partum period. The topics discussed were selected because they were believed to be pertinent to common obstetrical complications which matrones might be requested to treat. In conjunction with Professor Alihonou of the Faculty of Medicine, National University of Benin, questions were designed concerning frequently encountered obstetrical complications with which birth assistants in any culture would likely to be required to cope. Although questions were based on biomedical interpretations of labor and delivery, attempts were made to formulate descriptions of the biological concomitants of labor and delivery which were not culturally specific and could be recognized by matrones.

Questions were ordered following the chronology of the delivery process. Thus matrones were interviewed regarding estimated date of delivery; determination of fetal presentation (in order to evaluate modes of dealing with breech births, transverse presentations or other presentations); interpretations of normal and abnormal labor (in order to determine definitions of "complications" and reasons for calling a matrone); diagnosis of intrauterine death (in order to evaluate the range of diagnostic skills of matrones); treatment of the membranes (which has implications for likelihood of infection); treatment for delayed labor, fatigued parturients and numerous possible complications of labor such as: lacerations, bleeding, obstructed labor. Matrones were also asked to comment on post-partum complications with which they were familiar. The intent of this question was, again, to determine the complications most frequently encountered by matrones from amongst the complications which an obstetrician expects a specialist in obstetrics to encounter and the range of treatments employed in response to complications. Questions were in general intended to shed light on Bariba interpretations of a normal delivery, problematic delivery, and correspondingly, use of matrones.

(1) Date of Delivery: 11/12 matrones stated that they could not predict the date of delivery more accurately than by estimating the month of gestation. Some said a woman who was concerned about the date of delivery could consult a diviner or clairvoyant who might be able to predict the exact date of the onset of labor. Most women, however, do not bother.

(2) Perspective on Fetal Presentation: Of those matrones who responded, seven said that they had no means of checking the position of the baby prior

to delivery, while five respondents said that they did check. Those who claimed to determine the position of the baby varied in the means enabling verification. Two used palpation of the abdomen, stating that they could find the baby's head; one used internal examination; one observed the shape of the abdomen; and one relied on divination, using a special iron ring treated with herbs which enabled her to "see" inside the parturient.

(3) Inducing Labor: Of ten respondents, nine stated that they had no means of inducing labor. One matrone described cases of women who believed they were overdue (e.g., 12 months of pregnancy had passed) and said that she possessed a medicine to initiate labor in such situations. However, in spite of the fact that most women of reproductive age told stories about women who had overly long pregnancies, matrones generally did not treat this complaint.

(4) Average Length of Labor: Length of labor was determined to be a particularly salient topic because Bariba women often state that "long labor" is a reason for calling a matrone; moreover, dispensary and maternity clinic staff complain that women in labor often arrive seeking assistance "too late," after three or four days of obstructed labor. Perception of ideal length of labor was therefore a relevant consideration. In response to the question "how many times should the sun set on a woman in labor," most matrones commented that it is difficult to estimate length of labor because one is obliged to rely on the perceptions of the parturient herself. A complaining or fearful woman may divulge the fact that she is in labor after only a few contractions, whereas a courageous woman may never tell, or only after a day or even two, at which point she begins to be alarmed that labor is not progressing. In their response, 4/12 matrones thought "long labor" depended on the parturient, whether it was a primipara or multipara; two stated that two days of labor marked an excessively long labor; and two thought three days was overly long.

(5) Diagnosis of Intrauterine Death: Nine of eleven matrones stated that they were capable of judging fetal death. Basically, diagnosis was based on cessation of fetal movement or of contractions; either matrones interrogated the parturient and interpreted symptoms such as cessation of contractions, or observed and "felt" her abdomen in order to reach the conclusion of fetal death. In the event of intrauterine death, most matrones administered a medicine by mouth to accelerate contractions and cause the fetus to be expelled.

(6) Artificial Rupturing of Membrances: Of 13 matrones who responded to this question, eleven said that they never ruptured the membranes; this finding corresponded with the general observation that matrones rarely conduct vaginal examinations, measure cervical dilation, or touch the vagina area in any way. Some matrones explain their reluctance to conduct internal examinations by the fact that fingers inserted in the vaginal opening might injure the intestines of the parturient. The two who said that they did observed that sometimes the amniotic sac might be confused with "hemorrhoids" or other "protrusions" (i.e., *tigpiru*).

(7) Remedy for Fatigued Parturients: The most common remedy for exhaustion in a woman in labor was for the matrone to prepare an infusion for her, using leaves, bark or roots (5/12 respondents). Bark of the mustard tree (*Parkia biglobosa*) was one common treatment for fatigue. Two matrones rubbed pungent-smelling herbs on the stomach of the woman and held them under her nose to revive her. Two others used combinations of techniques – one infusion and a fumigation treatment and the other an incantation designed to revive the parturient.

(8) Accelerating a Delivery: Thirteen matrones (all who responded) agreed that they could accelerate a sluggish labor, by the same methods noted above; medicines to drink or ingest (such as mustard tree bark to chew) were particularly popular.

(9) Problems of Labor and Delivery: In discussing problems of labor which they had encountered, the following difficulties were mentioned: lacerations, cessation of contractions or lack of progression of labor, overly violent contractions, severe bleeding, and *tigpiru*. Most matrones had attempted to treat several of these complications and one elderly matrone said she had treated all of complications.

(10) Post-Partum Complications: Approximately half the matrones who responded (6/13) remained with the parturient for seven days in order to wash the baby, but the remainder waited only for the delivery of the placenta before departing. Nonetheless, nine noted post-partum complications with which they were familiar. These included hemorrhage, fever, breast abcess, and worms in the breast milk.

Overall, interviews with the matrones suggest similarities in problem definition in obstetrical cases. Although the exact choice of remedy may vary with each practitioner, (that is, which ingredients are used in a medicine, or whether gagging or pressure is preferred for a retained placenta, etc.) it is significant that more sorts of treatments were advocated for delivery of the ("retained") placenta than any other complication, which seems to indicate the importance attached to that condition. Retained placenta was in fact the most frequent reason for calling a matrone to a delivery, other than "long labor." Interviews with clients and observations of deliveries substantiated the use of the treatments described above. An additional very common treatment which matrones were relatively unified in advocating was fumigation for *tigpiru*, the "protruding" disease which is believed to inhibit delivery of the fetus and/or placenta. The contents of the fumigation mixture vary with each practitioner, however.

In sum, interviews with matrones, together with the case studies (some of which follow below) suggest that matrones share characteristics of style, technique and practice (see Table 13). Usually called in the event of complications, the matrone's first act is to observe the client for a while, often without touching her. Relatives who already attempted to help the parturient may explain length of labor, medicines administered, and significant symptoms. No matrones routinely do vaginal examinations. Depending on the problem, the matrone may:

(1) For "long labor," administer pungent-smelling herbs and massage the parturient's abdomen lightly; her thighs and back may also be rubbed but most matrones advise against it because the baby "is very near to the back" and those spots should not be touched for fear of harming the child;

(2) For "long labor" which does not respond to the above, a fumigation treatment for *tigpiru* or witchcraft will be tried, or

(3) Prepare a medicine to wash in, or

(4) Administer a medicine by mouth, in a preparation developed herself (by the matrone) but usually based on a preparation taught her by her mentor when she was an apprentice; matrones usually possess several treatments for less serious complications and probably one "special" medicine, to ingest, for severe complications;

(5) For retained placenta, administer medicine by mouth or fumigation and advise on use of the gagging stick or broom, which are therapies utilized by non-specialists as well;

TABLE 13
Techniques and practices of Bariba matrones

Techniques and practices	Number of matrones (Respondents/total respondents)
Could not estimate date of delivery	11/12
Don't verify fetal presentation	7/12
Don't induce labor	9/10
Can't diagnose intrauterine death	9/11
Don't rupture membranes	11/13
Have medicines for fatigued parturient	10/12
Can accelerate labor	13/13
Have treatment for retained placenta	14/14
Have treatment for *Tigpiru*	10/13

(6) Call a more experienced colleague to replace her if she is unable to treat the complication successfully. This colleague may be another matrone, or a male healer – either one who possesses an appropriate medicinal substance, and/or a ritual specialist such as the *gossiko* (burial official) who might better diagnose and treat the problem. If witchcraft is suspected or a witch baby diagnosed, the ritual specialist would then be a more appropriate one to deal with the situation.

Matrones may have additional cures which they have created – for in spite of the fact that there are many similarities in procedure, matrones would argue that each matrone *must* be different. If all were the same, who would be special?

That is why although matrones share concepts of causation of complications (e.g., witchcraft, *tigpiru*, adultery); definitions of complications (long labor, stillbirth, exhaustion, retained placenta); and notions of the available range of *types* of treatment, the therapy of choice and composition of the medicine remain the matrone's personal contribution to her professional practice.

Because matrones share certain concepts, techniques, and practices, it seems reasonable to assume that Bariba women expect the legimate practice of midwifery to fall within this range of concepts and behavior. Client expectations of a practitioner's proper behavior, then, will affect the selection of a healer, and predispose clients to select a matrone rather than a clinic.

CHAPTER 8

CLIENT-PRACTITIONER ENCOUNTERS

Perhaps the most illustrative approach to detailing the nature of the acceptable "range of therapeutic alternatives" is to present several cases of client-practitioner encounters. These cases will highlight some techniques, practices and concepts common to Bariba midwifery and will give an indication of the birth setting as well as of the characteristics of the relationship between the woman who is delivering and the matrone.

8.1.1. *The Case of Adama*

Previously, one common impetus for seeking a birth assistant was described as a situation where a woman experiences a problematic delivery. In the case of Adama Worou, the parturient, a woman in her late thirties or early forties and married to a Niger Djerma, came to the researcher to express her concern at feeling contractions when she was only eight months pregnant. Her worry over this occurrence was related to the belief that a baby born at eight months is a witch baby; whereas both a seven-month and a nine-month baby are normal children, an eight-month baby is referred to as a miscarriage and expected to die (or not to be allowed to live). However, many Bariba women are very vague in determining the expected date of delivery, which leads to some flexibility in interpreting the delivery of a witch baby. In this case, Adama initially claimed that she was in the eighth month of her pregnancy. Her attention to this detail may also have been related to the fact that she had a most worrisome reproductive history – twelve pregnancies and one child still living. She was, at the time of this delivery, newly married and pregnant for the first time by this husband. She was, then, very attentive to signs of another misfortune.

According to Adama, at 8 p.m. her contractions were not strong enough to prevent her from preparing the evening meal. She did stop by to visit the village nurse; he examined her and said her cervix was dilated to 4 cm. By 7 a.m. Adama sent someone to call me. When I arrived about 10 a.m., Adama was sitting on a mat, leaning on an elderly woman, her older brother's wife. The women were alone in the central room of a three-room house. The membranes had not yet broken and the old lady informed me that there was a while to wait. Meanwhile, she sat on a stool, pressing Adama's back where she complained of pain. (Other women advise parturients never to touch the back or the baby may be harmed; see, for example, the case of Bona.) Periodically the old lady said "God is," to Adama, who complained quietly, "wee, wee," a Bariba expression of pain.

At about 10:15, a Pehunko matrone, Yaayi Ganigi, appeared in the doorway, escorted by two Djerma-speaking elderly women of the husband's family.

Yaayi Ganigi sat down, ate some rice which was offered to her, and watched Adama. She did not examine her. She then told Adama to sit up and stop writhing – that twisting her body was bad for the baby. She told me that Adama was not yet ready to "push" because there wasn't any "water" standing out on her face, which would indicate imminence of delivery. Yaayi Ganigi asked the elderly women who were present if they had tried an application of certain pungent herbs. They had, but Ganigi asked for more; she rubbed Adama's stomach with water in which the leaves had been crushed, she held some of the wet leaves under her nostrils for her to smell, and rubbed her back on request. At 10:40, Adama got up and went into one of the adjoining rooms which had a bed in it, complaining that we were all looking at her. No one followed her or checked on her. Ganigi left the room (to tell the women outside to get the water ready, she later explained). Within five minutes, the baby was born, preceded immediately by the breaking of the membranes.

While awaiting the delivery of the placenta, Adama requested some porridge, which she drank. The household women brought the porridge-stirring stick to force in Adama's mouth. This is an extremely common method of inducing gagging which is intended to help expel the placenta. Yaayi Ganigi, however, turned down the offer of the stirring stick. Instead, she pushed on Adama's stomach a few times, told her to push, and used a straw broom, with which she rolled Adama's abdomen. When these techniques had no apparent effect, Ganigi took a special tiny gourd which she had brought, filled it with water and threw a needle into the gourd, with such force that it stuck in the gourd. Adama was then given the water to drink and the gourd was dropped on the baby, who was still lying on the floor. At this point, the baby was placed on a cloth. Ganigi then pulled on the cord lightly, at intervals, and finally burned some bark under Adama's vagina so that the smoke rose up. In all, these placenta-expelling attempts took about 12 minutes. Having exhausted her procedures, Ganigi and all the household women left the room, leaving me and Adama. I did not realize that I was expected to try my techniques now, following Ganigi's tacit withdrawal. In fact, because I saw some membrane delivered and the cord curl, I touched the cord slightly and the placenta was delivered, seemingly intact. Ganigi then returned and told me to cut the cord, which I declined to do, whereupon my lack of bravery was remarked on with some amusement. At 11:15, Ganigi cut the cord with a new razor blade. In order to cut it, she placed it on a millet stalk, and sliced it at her longest finger-length from the naval. She herself brought in a broken pot for the family to bury the placenta in the shower area behind the house, all the while complaining that Adama hadn't prepared anything for the baby's arrival (water jars, cloths).

Next, Ganigi washed the baby. A huge mound of soap was brought to her (*this* had been specially prepared for the baby). She cut off the top for herself as part of her compensation. She preceded to wash the baby and handed it over to the household women wrapped in a new cloth. At about 11:30, Ganigi's niece Zenabu and her co-wife arrived to congratulate Adama, who was still in the bedroom. Then, Adama went to wash herself with hot water and potash and butter soap and thereafter, to receive more visitors.

The following day, I went to call on Yaayi Ganigi, in order to ask why Adama's family had called Ganigi when some women delivered alone. Ganigi replied: "You yourself saw how she behaved, twisting and turning. A woman like that could kill the child if no old lady were with her."

8.1.1.1. *Comments*

Some points surface in the unfolding of this case which require additional consideration.

(1) The eight-month pregnancy. It seems that the decision to call for assistance was based on two factors: (a) suspected prematurity, indicating witchcraft, and (b) a reproductive history fraught with misfortune. It is interesting that no mention was made of the prematurity of the baby after Adama's initial private comment to me. This might be the result of various factors – possibly, I was the only person to whom Adama mentioned her concern because others might not have kept close count and be able to confront her with this fact. She herself was very worried about delivering and keeping the baby, especially in light of her reproductive history. The women of the household were aware of her numerous infant losses, however. At the moment of delivery, a discussion arose as to whether to call the child "Yo." When a mother has had several children die, the one who is born following the deaths may be called "slave," or "Yo." In this event, the attendants figuratively sell the child to a stranger, neighbor or relative so that it is no longer the child of its cursed mother. Until the age of 10 or so, a "Yo" will take gifts to its "owner" and wear its hair half-shaved in the manner of a slave. (There are also other ways of trying to safeguard a child born of a mother whose children die – one is to yell at the child and tell it the earth is full, there is no ground to bury it in; another is to tie a string from one arm, across the baby's back, to the other arm, to "attach" it to life, or to have the child wear iron anklets, symbolizing its attachment to the earth and life.) In the case of Adama, her brother's wife decided that it was not necessary to name the child "Yo" because it was the first delivery by a new husband; the dead children had all belonged to a previous spouse. The final decision was that nothing had to be done immediately. Thus it seems likely that given the successful delivery, the option to declare the child a witch was not taken.

(2) During her labor, Adama cooked dinner, in conformity with the value placed on women continuing their household work and ignoring (or pretending to ignore) contractions. Later, however, Adama did express pain, and complained particularly of back pains. Although the matrone and Adama's brother's wife were sympathetic and did rub her back, others were critical of this indulgence. It is also noteworthy that the matrone, in conversation after the delivery, described Adama as fearful and commented disapproving on her twisting and turning. As an observer who has attended deliveries in an American hospital and deliveries in Benin of non-Bariba who are less concerned with stoicism, I

did not think Adama "twisted and turned" excessively and she was very quiet; her expressions of "wee" were infrequent and low-pitched. The degree of expression which is necessary to label a person as uncontrolled and fearful seems very low indeed.

(3) The matrone, Yaayi Ganigi, did not examine the parturient internally; her evaluation of the stage of labor was apparently based on visual appraisal of Adama's appearance. The amniotic sac was not broken and no one asked about it except me. The answer to a question regarding the breaking of the membranes is invariably that the "water of delivery" (*soomo*) never breaks unless the delivery is imminent; if one sees water but the baby doesn't follow, the liquid was not the true "water of delivery."

(4) In accordance with the belief that the placenta should be delivered immediately following the baby, the household women galvanized into action, bringing an object to induce gagging and the matrone attempted various efforts designed to expel the placenta. When none of these efforts were successful, the women left the room, expecting me to try my remedies. This is the classical procedure in healing, wherein one healer tries a cure, fails, leaves, and another arrives. It is rare for spectators to observe a healer, thus I was left unobserved.

(5) Regarding the matrone herself, she is in an aristocratic Bariba woman in her 60's, trained in midwifery by her mother-in-law; she is married to a wealthy Hausa trader (her second marriage – the first was to a Bariba aristocrat) and lives in the neighborhood of Zongo. Zongo residents are primarily "foreigners," Dendi, Djerma, and Hausa-speaking. Yaayi Ganigi speaks Dendi and Hausa and serves as the principal midwifery resource for Zongo. Adama's household is located in Zongo neighborhood, and the husband's female relatives speak Dendi. They communicated with the matrone in Dendi. My impression is that many of Ganigi's clients are women who have links to Ganigi's husband, either themselves or through their own husbands, and her ability to communicate in the languages of the "foreigners" is considered a great asset by the Zongo population.

8.1.2. *The Case of Sako*

The case of Sako, another client of Yaayi Ganigi, illustrates symptom interpretation and an instance of referral. Sako, pregnant with her second child, was the Bariba wife of a Hausa neighbor of Yaayi Ganigi. The first had been born in another village. Here, one would note that Sako is under 4′10″ in height, and in western medicine would be considered a high-risk patient because of her size. Sako went to see Yaayi Ganigi in the late afternoon to complain of pain. Ganigi asked her if it were the 10th (lunar) month, which it was. Ganigi took her to an empty storage room (Ganigi is one of the few matrones who ever has clients who deliver at her house, rather than calling her to come to them) where she "pushed" for several hours. According to Ganigi, Sako did not want to open her legs or to remove her skirt which provoked Ganigi to tell her "I've seen many women at birth, women worth a lot more than you!" Finally, because the baby seemed high in her stomach, Ganigi suggested that Sako consult the village nurse at the dispensary.

Sako went to the dispensary, accompanied by her co-wife and several elderly female relatives of her husband. At the dispensary, the nurse said that Sako was fully dilated and told her to lie on the table. She refused, saying that she could not push and that the child would rise up into her throat rather than descend if she lay down. As at the matrone's, she refused to remove her skirt and persisted in sitting on the floor with her legs stretched in front of her, one crossed over the other. When told to walk around by the old ladies who had accompanied her, she refused. For the most part, one old lady stayed with Sako while the others waited outside. The nurse gave her the pungent herbs to smell which are much-relied upon by matrones, as well as two injections, with no apparent progress of labor. Finally, the old lady rubbed the herbs on her stomach and sent home for a medicine to drink. While this medicine was administered, the nurse was outside the building. The old lady, after each rubbing gesture on Sako's stomach, tapped her fingers on the floor. After giving Sako the medicine to drink, she dropped the gourd on the floor (symbolizing the dropping of the child). Significantly, the matrone Ganigi was not called back, in spite of the obvious conclusion that the nurse's medicine was not effective. The husband's old lady, although not known as a matrone, seemed to have some skills and to be confident that her remedies were appropriate.

By 10 p.m., Sako still was fully dilated, not pushing, and sitting silently on the floor with her legs crossed. Finally, Bata, the president of women of Pehunko (titled *yaayikpe*), dropped by to check on the delivery. A tall, heavy woman, Bata dragged Sako to her knees, and placed her in the "proper" position for delivery as the nurse watched. The husband's old lady gave Sako another drink, in which fragments resembling purple fruit peel were floating. Bata then told two of the assembled women to come in and hold Sako's legs apart. Shortly thereafter, she delivered a stillborn child with a misshapen head. The women were silent; the nurse told Sako she had killed the baby.

8.1.2.1. *Comments*

Both the matrone and the attending women were confused by the apparent lack of descent of the baby; all the women observed that Sako's stomach was "high" and that a bump could be felt at the fundus whereas no bump could be felt in the lower abdominal region. In actuality, there was no "bump" at the pubic level because the head was already in the pelvis. Because the women assumed delivery was not imminent, they refused to urge Sako to push. However, they did react with disapproval to her refusing to uncross her legs or walk around and some attributed the stillborn child to this behavior. In discussion regarding this delivery, one woman commented that Sako's own family probably would not talk about this misfortune or criticize Sako to her face. However, her equals (friends, women her age) would bring up the subject in an argument about something else (for example, if Sako were to act arrogantly, someone might reply "you should talk, at your delivery you behaved badly . . . " and she would be ashamed). Although I could not get anyone to confirm my suspicion, I suspect that Sako had either broken a taboo, committed adultery or had some private reason to dread the delivery of the child – either, as is the procedure in adultery, she would need to confess the name of the adulterer or she could not deliver, or she feared she had done something which would cause the child to be abnormal. For this reason, she refused to uncross her legs, either for a matrone or the nurse.

Other than the implications for social control indicated in this case (adultery, gossip, shaming by age-cohorts) it is interesting to note the simultaneous utilization of western medicine and indigenous medicine. Sako began by consulting a matrone (possibly at the urging of her husband, a Hausa, or due to her fears, of whatever origin). The matrone administered Bariba medicines and referred her to the nurse. The nurse gave her injections and herbs which act as smelling salts, and told her to wait. Thereupon, the discontented family gave her massage and medicine by mouth. Finally, a visiting (and prestigious) friend took charge of the psychological support functions of the situation, while the nurse tried to manoeuver the delivery of the head, complicated by the swelling. The nurse claimed with annoyance that when several people administer treatments, the one who gave the last therapy prior to the delivery gets credit for success, even if "physiology" is really explanation for the outcome. In this case, however, no one received credit for success, even though the mother's life was saved. The nurse thought that the mother had inhibited a spontaneous, easier delivery, the women also thought Sako had inhibited her labor and behaved shamefully, although their medicines had contributed to making the best of a bad situation. The matrone thought Sako was stubborn, and Sako never commented on what she thought.

8.1.3. *The Case of the Prolapsed Cord*

This case clearly illustrates how interpretation of symptoms and subsequent action designed to alleviate these symptoms are based on culturally derived expectations which define the problem at hand. In this instance, Ganigi, in the late stages of her 10th pregnancy (exact week or month unknown) called her mother and complained that "something had come out of her vagina." Because of the modesty which obtains between mother and daughter, the mother did not examine the protruding object; nor was anyone else available in the household who might have felt in a position to regard the pregnant woman's genital area. Instead, the mother of the woman sent a messenger to a matrone, Yaayi Bore, the first wife of the former village chief, and a woman noted for her spiritual powers and healing abilities. The messenger was instructed to inform Bore of the problem, in other words, to request a treatment for dealing with a protruding object which was considered abnormal. Bore herself did not visit the pregnant women; rather, she responded to the description of the problem, which she immediately defined as *tigpiru*.

Tigpiru was described in chapter 2 as a condition characterized by lower abdominal pain or back pain. It is considered to be an internal growth which, as the illness progresses, becomes red, takes a round form "like an egg," and protrudes through the anus or vagina. If the illness does not protrude, it may lie flat in the abdomen and cause swollen legs and feet. *Tigpiru* is a common explanation for swollen legs, ankles and feet during pregnancy. According to the nurses and nurse-midwives with whom I discussed this condition, when Bariba speak of *tigpiru* they are probably referring variably to hemorrhoids, prolapsed uterus, cystoceles, or rectoceles.[26]

Women complain that this is the most common female disorder and most matrones possess medicines to treat it. The usual procedure is for a woman to take a preventive medicine during the last month of pregnancy to cause the obstruction to shrink and rise up in her body. If left untreated, the obstacle will obstruct labor or inhibit the delivery of the placenta. In the event of a slow labor or retained placenta which is believed to be due to *tigpiru*, the matrones have two treatments of choice – one is a product taken by mouth with some porridge; the other is treatment by fumigation. In the fumigation method, the medicine (which appears to be a mixture of dried grasses) is placed on a piece of broken pottery or tin, on top of burning coals. As it smolders, it is held under the woman's vagina so that the smoke will rise and cause any obstruction to dissipate.

In this case, having diagnosed a severe case of *tigpiru* in which the illness had progressed to its external stage and had fallen completely out of the vagina (it should be remembered that until this point, no one except the pregnant woman herself had actually looked at the protrusion), Yaayi Bore, the matrone, sent over a fumigation mixture of cotton, bark and grasses to be burnt under the woman's vagina. The end-result which was sought was for the obstruction to rise back up and send the child back to its correct place or if it was another illness, to cause it to come out completely in the form of water. However, it did nothing. At this point, the woman's family sent for the researcher and the village nurse. In the absence of the nurse, I went. When the woman's mother informed me of the problem, and told me she had not looked at the "obstruction" due to embarrassment, I looked and saw immediately that it was a section of the umbilical cord, indicating a prolapsed cord. Because of the possibility of fetal suffering which a prolapsed cord may signify, I suggested that we evacuate the woman to the nearest maternity clinic.

The family consulted and decided to call a second matrone, Yaayi Yo, a neighbor and distant relation to the parturient's mother. Yo came in person, checked the cord and suggested that the objective should be to induce the obstruction to protrude further so we could examine it and better identify it. At this point, she, I and the nurse's apprentice were present; the woman's mother again left the room. Yo first administered pungent herbs to smell, hoping to induce contractions. She also lightly massaged the woman's abdomen with these same herbs. Next she left and returned with a gourd full of a liquid which she instructed the woman to drink. Shortly thereafter, the woman's abdomen could be seen to ripple wih a contraction. But after this one visible contraction, no other effect could be observed. Periodically during the treatment, I had suggested that the protrusion was the umbilical cord and the woman should be transported to the district clinic. Eventually, I altered my explanation and said that a piece of the placenta was protruding. Evidently the sight of the cord did not remind her of an umbilical cord, perhaps because in her obstetrical experiences, she had never seen such a sight. When I suggested it was the placenta, Yo responded thoughtfully that sheep sometimes deliver the placenta before the lamb (this remark was consistent with the matrone Yo's approach to healing via understanding animals. In another instance, she explained miscarriages by comparison with baby mice.) The nurse's apprentice then interrupted to remind the matrone that women are not sheep and the mother, pregnant woman, other females of the household and the matrone assembled to discuss the most appropriate action to take.

The pregnant woman cried because she was sure the protruding cord was "abnormal," and possibly indicated a dangerous child who was trying to kill her. The matrone, who was in general very opposed to cosmopolitan medical services, demurred at the idea of sending the woman to the district maternity clinic. The nurse's apprentice argued in support of sending her, and eventually the family agreed. They chose a young cousin to accompany her on the trip. Upon arrival at the clinic, the nurse-midwife determined that the prolapsed cord was associated with twins, the first of which (a boy) was stillborn and in a transverse presentation. Both twins were delivered vaginally (without any anesthetic) and the second, a girl, seemed healthy, although very tiny. The family explained the situation *ex post facto* by saying that the first twin wanted to kill its mother but was prevented by me. My understanding of the problem was believed to have been gained by placing my hand on the woman's stomach which I did at one point while still at her home, in an attempt to gauge the position of the fetus, and *not* by my observing the protruding cord. (Quote overheard after the delivery, in reference to myself: all that she [the researcher] did was *touch* her stomach and she knew immediately what was wrong!)

8.1.3.1. *Comments*

There are two points regarding the selection of a matrone which are noteworthy here. As in other cases, the matrone was called due to the appearance of an abnormality, the prolapsed cord. When the first matrone, Bore, provided a medicine which did not work, the family did not call her back in order to request a different medicine or to ask the matrone's opinion. Rather, they tried a second matrone. They asked my advice first, but my immediate response to transport the woman to the district clinic was found disagreeable, and Yo was called. When I became involved, I tried to enlist Bore's help in order to avoid assuming full responsibility myself, but Bore refused to come unless I said I couldn't do anything and that the case was beyond my powers. However, the family did not ask her again. I tried to address this issue directly by asking the parturient's mother why she called Bore first but didn't ask her advice when the *tigpiru* fumigation yielded no results. The mother replied that (1) she had called Bore first because "Bore is known everywhere for her powers, she is even written about in books!" (2) Second, she called Yaayi Yo because Yo works "together with Bore." This second statement sounded very tantalizing, but further investigation provided no support for the contention that the two worked together. They had never been known to be present simultaneously at a delivery; they are not kin, and although both belong to the *sambani* possession cult, they participate in different branches. I concluded that the two matrones probably do not work together and that the parturient's mother was merely trying to avoid criticizing the lack of success of Yaayi Bore's treatment.

At the beginning of this case, I suggested it as an illustration of the relationship of a selection of a treatment to interpretation of symptoms and to expectations regarding the problem at hand. It is worth re-emphasizing this point. The prolapsed cord was diagnosed as a prevalent folk syndrome (*tigpiru*); the fact that it did not completely conform to the characteristics of *tigpiru* (i.e., it was not round and red) was overlooked (a) because it was a protrusion from the vagina, also a sign of *tigpiru* and (b) because of the cultural prohibitions on the mother viewing her daughter's genitals. Both these factors – diagnosis of *tigpiru* and modesty – are associated with the hesitation of the women in this case to use the maternity clinic. Bariba women in general share this reluctance to use national health clinics if *tigpiru* is suspected.

First, *tigpiru* is considered prevalent among Bariba women but it is assumed that Europeans and government health personnel do not understand this condition, cannot diagnose it, and hence will not treat it. This is borne out by the treatment of swollen feet in the government maternity clinic. When women go for prenatal care to the district clinic (and also for those few who visit the village nurse), their feet and shins are checked for signs of oedema. In the event that swelling is observed, the nurse or nurse-midwife invariably advises the woman not to eat salt, so that the swelling will subside. Most women receiving this advice do not think that it is relevant to curing swollen feet, which is believed to be due to *tigpiru* and require fumigation treatments for alleviation of the condition. It is clear, then, why the woman and her relatives, faced with the prolapsed cord, did not panic or take immediate action to consult a nurse; even more than the usual hesitations, the diagnosis of a folk condition precluded utilization of a modern service and therapist within whose realm of competence the condition did not fall. (Even though a majority of women do not attend clinics or dispensaries for prenatal care, the advice or "taboo" regarding salt has become well-known throughout the region. Even Yaayi Bore, the elderly matrone, who does not reside near a clinic nor accept clinic utilization as a satisfactory alternative for obstetrical care, mentioned, unsolicited, the warning of nurses not to eat salt.)

8.1.4. *The Case of the Terrifying Breech*

This case illustrates the personality attributes useful to the matrone in performing her role satisfactorily. The story was recounted by Yon Sika of Doh as an example of the most frightening event of her professional life, and in fact, the worst thing she ever saw.

Do you know the worst thing I ever saw, she asked? (Chorus of listening women: what?) It was a baby. (Chorus: what kind of baby?) It was a woman who had been in labor for several days when they called me. I gave her some medicine to drink so that she would push; then when she was kneeling, I saw the terrible sight. It was the buttocks of the baby appearing first [in the vagina]. I wanted to leave the room but the woman begged me to stay with her so I did. When the baby fell, it was delivered *sitting up*. (The fate of this child is unknown; from exclamations of horror by the audience, one might surmise that the child was not allowed to live.)

The matrone continued: I became as white as a Fulani cheese from fear. Later, I became ill from what I had seen and had to consult an old man who cured me. That was the worst sight I have ever seen.

8.1.4.1. *Comments*

In this case, it is clear that the matrone needed the qualities of courage and fortitude, as well as compassion for the parturient in order to stay with her during the delivery and to restrain herself from fleeing the terrible sight of the breech presentation. The matrone Yon Sika is in fact known throughout the village of Doh for her charitable nature, in comparison with the other practicing matrone, who is not always willing to come to a delivery when called. It is also noteworthy that Yon Sika as the assisting matrone was herself endangered by the sight of the abnormal birth. She actually became ill from the sight and was obliged to undergo a curative treatment to restore her "health." A matrone, then, always risks this kind of ordeal and requires both prophylactic medicine to fortify herself against the risks and personal attributes to sustain her while performing her function.

8.1.5. *The Case of Bona*

The following case exemplifies the classic case of a woman who has always delivered easily and alone, but finds herself in a problematic situation and decides to call for assistance. The case also illustrates the midwifery procedures favored by a third matrone of Pehunko, Yaayi Bore, the matrone who provided the fumigation medicine for the woman with the prolapsed cord. At this delivery, the parturient (Bona) was expecting her fourth child. In part because of her friendship with the researcher, she had attended prenatal consultations with a visiting obstetrician from the capital and had also consulted once with the village nurse regarding cramps in her legs. Bona said she felt contractions during the night but in the morning, she said nothing and sold beans as usual while the other women went to the fields. At noon, a child was sent to ask for my assistance because Bona was worried due to the nurse's prediction that she would deliver twins. (The nurse was out-of-town.) Bona walked to the dispensary where she learned that the nurse was really absent, and then called for her older sister. The older sister decided to call Bore, the chief's wife and neighbor of Bona's father-in-law's household. Meanwhile, Bona requested that I bring the medicines to accelerate delivery which the old matrone of Doh, Sika, had given me. I was not immediately obliged to decide on the ethics of administering the powders because Bona's mother-in-law returned from the fields and told Bona to wait for Bore before taking any action.

Finally Bore arrived with a gourd and three small medicine containers. She touched Bona's lower back, asked her if she wanted to push and if the water of delivery had come yet. Bona replied negatively to both questions and Bore pronounced her not ready to deliver yet. Bore gave the sister medicine to heat in water; Bona had gone to urinate in the shower and stayed there so Bore took her the medicine to drink. Following administration of the medicine, she dropped the gourd in the gesture that symbolizes the falling of the child. Next Bore told the mother-in-law and Bona to move from the mat on which we were sitting into another room without a ceiling; the room with a ceiling provoked fear in her "because the ceiling thinks it is a chief," so we moved to a storage room. Next Bore prayed, washing her hands and feet, in a corner of the courtyard and then prepared a fumigation medicine (*duku*) in case some obstruction was inhibiting Bona's labor from progressing. Bona sat over the smoldering coals for about three minutes (she said it was hot). Her contractions seemed to increase (judging from observation of the surface of her abdomen). Periodically, Bona went off to the shower area behind the house, possibly to obtain some privacy. No one commented when she left.

During one of her departures, the matrone took me to look for a certain insect's nest which is laid on the dirt walls of houses. I found one and cut it off the wall for her. She then crushed it, mixed it with water and rubbed it on Bona's stomach in semi-circular motions, to the right and to the left. Subsequently (laughing and telling the family in the courtyard that I was her assistant) she took me to find a mustard tree (*Parkia biglobosa*) to cut off some bark. I carried the bark for her, the proper role for a subordinate; she then peeled it and gave some to Bona to chew (the fiber is spit out and the juice is swallowed.) By this time about an hour and a half had passed and Bore left. Bona told me that this delivery was much worse than her others and she was worried. She asked again for "my" medicines (from Doh) but Bore then returned with another medicine to drink. The gourd was dropped again with the exclamation "*baraka*" which is said when the child is delivered. Shortly thereafter, Bona began to kneel because she felt like pushing. Her back hurt and she wanted to lean forward but Bore told her not to touch her back because the child was close to the skin there during pregnancy and to sit up straight.

Bore supported her from behind while she was kneeling and briefly, her older sister was called to do so. Prior to the delivery of the baby, the amniotic sac became visible. I asked if it could be broken but Bore said no and prepared another fumigation medicine to deal with this obstacle. Before she could do so, it burst and the baby was born. Immediately Bore tugged on the cord and told the sister to get a scarf. This scarf was held taut and used to massage Bona's stomach to expel the placenta. Another female relative (the husband's father's brother's wife) arrived with a porridge-stick to induce gagging. The matrone told me to push on her stomach but I (alarmed over the pulling on the cord) suggested waiting. After two minutes, the placenta was delivered; it seemed to be missing a segment and in fact Bona lost a couple pots full of blood. Bore promptly left.

The father's brother's wife came to cut the cord, first marking the spot with sandstone, then placing the cord against a millet stalk and cutting it with a new blade. Some debate occurred over the best place to cut the cord; the cord-cutter prevailed in her decision to measure the cord against the right knee of the baby. The cord stump bled, so the cord-cutter spit chewed charcoal on it and friends appeared immediately to "greet" the baby. Bona went to wash herself and the cord-cutter proceeded to wash the baby.

The baby washing ritual occurred in one of its more thorough versions. The washer scrubbed the baby twice with a fibre sponge and potash and butter soap, rinsing it in "*koru*," a special water made from the water left when shea butter is prepared and saved for the first washing of a baby. This butter water is designed to remove "the blood" of the delivery from the child. After the washing, the baby was buttered with shea butter, including her anus, and pressed. Her nose was pushed up to the forehead to prevent its being flat and then raised in relief. Then her head was pressed in from both sides and from both ends so that a fold could be seen along the back of the head when pressed sideways. Three or four times the arms were pressed palm up and palm down and stretched out. The legs were similarly handled. The washer then crossed the baby's legs behind it and pushed her body down, her lower back was pushed in, her chest pushed hard enough so that finger marks showed. She was then held in the air by the hands and shaken, shaken lightly upside down and tossed three times in the air (with her head held firmly) to give her courage. Finally, another of the husband's relatives helped perfume and dress the baby, put antimony on her eyes and eyebrows and wrap her in some cloths.

Meanwhile, Bona had begun to worry that she was bleeding excessively and expressed her concern to me. I suggested (in the absence of any appropriate drugs or competent diagnostician) that she stop walking around, lie down and place ice on her abdomen. The women of the household, particularly her mother-in-law and the father-in-law's brother's wife relieved her fears by telling her that bleeding is therapeutic and cleanses the stomach of impurities, *tigpiru*, dysmenorrhea (painful menstruation), etc. Several hours later, when the bleeding continued to a degree that the women thought unhealthy, they called the nurse's apprentice (Bona had by then drunk the ice which I intended as an ice pack) who gave Bona an injection of a "heart stimulant" (syncortyl). The bleeding slowed down without further intervention and by evening, Bona was eating porridge and milk prepared for her by her husband's sister. This same sister also prepared the preferred sauce for post-partum diet, which is composed of nuts (*dukubinu*) and bark (*tabu*) imported from Nigeria, mustard, condiments, and green leaves. This sauce is intended to "help the blood come out."

The following day, Bona complained of extreme cramps, in spite of the sauces she had eaten which are intended to alleviate such discomfort. (It is retained blood which causes pain; the sauce acts, then, by stimulating the blood to flow out.) Bona asked me if any of my "old ladies" (matrones) had given me a medicine to treat these pains. I recommended a certain sauce advocated by the matrone from Doh. This sauce contained: *dukubinu* nuts, *tabu* bark, pepper and crushed leaves known as "*swadobarakaru*." While she was preparing this sauce for herself, an elderly woman who lived next door passed by and asked Bona how she was feeling. Bona complained of her cramps and the old woman recommended the same sauce. Bona thanked her but did not tell her she already knew about it. After eating the sauce, she claimed she felt much better and explained that her pains were probably due to the injection which the nurse's apprentice had given her the day before. (According to the Bariba interpretation, by cutting off the bleeding, the injection had caused pain because pain is prevented by bleeding, thus eliminating the pain agent with blood.)

8.1.5.1. *Comments*

During the course of Bona's delivery, therapies from differing medical traditions were opted for alternatively.

(1) Bona attended prenatal consultations with a visiting obstetrican and the village nurse.

(2) She requested that the researcher, nurse, and her older sister assist her at her delivery.

(3) In the absence of the nurse, she chose (based on her sister's advice) a local matrone, a neighbor.

(4) While waiting for the matrone to arrive and when the matrone's treatments seemed ineffective, she asked the researcher to administer a Bariba medicine acquired during the researcher's apprenticeship in another village.

(5) When Bona experienced excessive bleeding post-partum, she contacted:

   (a) The researcher, whose advice was overruled by,
   (b) The mother-in-law and father-in-law's brother's wife, whose opinion was swayed by the duration of the bleeding and who called,
   (c) The nurse's apprentice who injected Bona with a drug not specifically indicated for the condition.

This variety of treatment seem to indicate a pragmatic interest on the part of the parturient and her relatives in coping with complications as they arose. The alternative and consecutive use of indigenous and cosmopolitan services suggests the difficulty in characterizing people's preferences for birth assistance, and in general, medical treatment (See also Colson 1971; Fabrega 1978). The intermingling of western medical and indigenous Bariba obstetrical practices is also much in evidence in deliveries which occurred in the Pehunko dispensary, although less so in the district maternity clinic, where the nurse-midwives tend to be more authoritative in maintaining their "preserve."

Also of note in this case were the symbolic gestures used by the matrone, Bore, in the course of her ministerings. One such gesture was the application of the crushed insect larva to Bona's abdomen. This procedure was later interpreted by several matrones as representing a successful delivery. The preference is to a particular insect, which is said to not produce offspring itself; it merely builds a house on the wall (*kpansa*) around a larva (its offspring) and the offspring bursts out. The matrone represents the insect, drawing out an offspring which is not from her own body. Similarly, the matrone on two occasions administered medicines to drink from a gourd and then dropped the gourd to symbolize the dropping of the child, and exemplifying the principle of "contagious magic" inherent in much of Bariba medicine.

A final point which is raised in this delivery involves the question of the solitary delivery. At all the deliveries which were observed or on which information was obtained immediately post-partum, immediately upon delivery of the child, even if the woman delivered completely alone, someone came almost instantaneously to cut the umbilical cord and to check on the delivery of the placenta. Then neighbors appeared to congratulate the mother and greet the child. This consistent appearance of a cord-cutter and of the neighbors suggests that although the parturient may be physically alone during the delivery, family and friends are aware of the situation and are unobtrusively following all stages of labor and delivery (at least to the extent that others can guess by certain signs that a woman is in labor) and are ready to appear at the last act to provide a chorus of salutations. In this sense, a delivery is a performance and cannot be considered as a purely individual and solitary act.

8.2. PAIN AS A CULTURAL PHENOMENON

Throughout the observation of deliveries, the lack of expression of pain or discomfort by women in labor was striking especially to an observer with experience in maternity wards in other cultures, such as the United States and southern Benin. This behavioral response common to Bariba women during childbirth seems worthy of further discussion regarding the interpretation of the responses observed. Bariba women almost never uttered any verbal expression of pain other than softly clicking their teeth or muttering "wee" under their breath. Most made no sounds at all, including the woman with the prolapsed cord, who had a stillborn child turned internally and removed without anesthetic. In the above presentation of cases, mention was made of Adama, who from the researcher's perspective, could hardly have been called a complainer or hysterical but who was scorned by the matrone for twisting her body all around, in an uncontrolled manner harmful to the baby. One might speculate, then, that the cultural criteria regarding the appropriate responses to pain seem to necessitate self-discipline and stoicism, regardless of discomfort.

In trying to further interpret the reactions of Bariba women in childbirth, it becomes evident that the literature on pain includes few references to the influence of culture on response to pain (Wolff and Langley 1968:494). Wolff and Langley, in their review of the literature on this subject, note that investigations of the Pain Group of the Department of Medicine of NYU Medical Center showed a difference in pain response due to ethnocultural factors. In general, the authors state that experimental studies do not allow a definite conclusion on whether basic differences in pain response exist among ethnic groups but there is strong evidence that they do (499). Unfortunately, few studies have been undertaken where the experimenters were skilled in the application of experimental pain-inducing techniques, and specifically investigated cultural or ethnic effects on pain response (Wolff and Langley 1968:498).[27]

The available data on Bariba responses to labor and delivery also lacks the element of rigorous controlled measurement of pain intensity and response. However, the data do shed light on the extent to which learning and experience shape perceptions of pain and behavior of persons in pain (cf. Fabrega and Tyma 1976b). Behavioral responses are not necessarily correlated with the intensity of the pain *sensation*. Studies on the measurement of pain intensity in childbirth have demonstrated that

> The reactions of the patient depend partly on the pain and to a greater extent on fatigue, anxiety, and in some cases hostility . . . whereas pain intensity as measured was related to the uterine activity and dilation of the cervical and perineal tissues. It seems important, therefore, to make a clear distinction between the intensity of the pain perceived by the patient and visible evidences of reaction to pain, such as complaining, groaning and crying out. (Hardy and Javert 1949:161)

The intensity of pain, then, cannot always be evaluated by the reaction or correlated with the manifestation of distress. In the classic anthropological study of the cultural dimensions of pain, Zborowski postulated that there is no such phenomenon as a "natural" physiological function (e.g., pain) which is not shaped by cultural influences and suggested that " . . . the 'cultural' nature of physiological activities implies that they have to be learned, not only on the level of reflex conditioning, but also on the level of interpersonal relationships, through words and example." (Zborowski 1969: 21–22). According to Zborowski, people respond to pain as members of an ethnic group, hence there is a sociocultural dimension to pain, distinct from the psychological or physiological interpretation (21).[28]

One might ask, however, if it is not possible that for some reason, childbirth is less painful to Bariba women than to women in other cultures (cf. Freedman and Ferguson 1950). Freedman and Ferguson concluded in their article on this subject that "it has been empirically demonstrated that the pain of childbirth can be diminished and in some cases eliminated by the application of suitable techniques, even of a rather simple and superficial nature." But, they caution, " . . . at least in the case of the pain of childbirth, the fact that agony may be increased or decreased by environmental manipulation should not blind us to the physiological actuality of its sources or the universality of its existence" (Freedman and Ferguson 1950:370–371).

It is interesting that the argument of Freedman and Ferguson closely parallels the perspective of the majority of Bariba women with whom the subject was discussed. First, the question of the reality of pain in childbirth was proposed to women; that is, it was suggested to them that the reason women often seemed expressionless and did not complain during delivery was because they were not experiencing pain or discomfort. This was denied categorically by both parturients and matrones. One matrone, Yon Sika, commented that this same issue is sometimes raised when Bariba women travel to other regions, for example, following husbands engaged in commerce in Nigeria. If the Bariba woman delivers in the presence of other women of neighboring ethnic groups, the parturient or her husband are likely to be asked to share whatever medicine they have which prevents the parturient from feeling pain and permits her to maintain such control. The matrone Yon Sika suggested that women do not show pain because a woman who did so would "eat shame" and never be allowed to forget her lack of self-discipline and her cowardice. This matrone also noted that while she did not have a medicine to take away *pain*, she did have a medicine to take away *fear*. It is the effect of fear which causes women to be unable to remain controlled, to cry out or twist their bodies unseemingly or to ask for help. When a fearful woman eats this medicine, she may feel the same degree of pain, but she will be able to overcome it. One school of thought holds that the experiencing of pain is lessened when the individual manages to control the manifestation or responses to it but this possibility could not be addressed in the present research project. A similar statement was put forth by the matrone Gingire [Soaodou] who possessed a medicine invented by her husband. This medicine was designed for the same purpose as that described above. In addition, it came in two forms – a product to wash in for women, and one to take in the form of snuff for men. (A warning accompanies this medicine: it must be taken in moderation; too much makes a person lose perspective and become brazen.)

Matrones claim that it is very difficult to determine that a properly controlled woman is actually ready to deliver. It requires an experienced observer to do so; one sign is known as "the language of feet," and refers to the clenching of toes of a woman in labor. Even a stoical woman will give herself away by this sign. Sweat on the face is also considered an indicator by some. Curiously, although most women are very reluctant to express pain during labor, many women will complain about post-partum discomfort and will request of others a medicine to alleviate this pain. Thus the focus of the effort to remain impassive and controlled seems to be the actual labor and delivery and to be somewhat lessened post-partum.

Referring again to Zborowski's study of responses to pain, one finds additional comments which illuminate an interpretation of the behavior of Bariba women. Zborowski (1969:19) lists five behavior responses to pain. These include:

(1) motor responses (e.g., twisting, clenching teeth);
(2) vocal responses (e.g., screaming, moaning);
(3) verbal responses (e.g., cursing, complaining);
(4) social responses (e.g., change in manners, withdrawal);
(5) absence of manifest behavior (e.g., hiding of pain or suppressing extreme signs of pain).

Based on observed deliveries and reports by matrones and nurse-midwives, the most common behavioral response to childbirth by Bariba women is the fifth item, "absence of manifest behavior." As Zborowski underscores, cultural traditions dictate correct conduct during a pain experience (32). Correspondingly, a consideration of other occurrences affecting both Bariba men and women, in which pain might be experienced suggests that the deprecation of pain and the conception that lack of self-discipline reflects cowardice and merits shame, are common to other situations than childbirth. Bravery in war and hunting and stoicism in the event of injuries incurred in those activities is greatly admired among men; even in the event of an injury such as a scorpion bite, a person is expected to try not to tell anyone he has been bitten and to continue with normal work (nonetheless, the typical description of a scorpion bit is that it keeps the victim awake all night with throbbing pain.) Children are also expected to behave bravely but are not scorned for cowardice as are adults; almost all girls cry during the female circumcision ceremony, for example. (Male circumcision is done on babies.)

The Pehunko village dispensary was a useful setting in which to observe reactions to pain and anxiety. The primary form of treatment at the dispensary was an injection; injections are vastly preferred by patients and are believed to more effective than tablets or syrups. They are also considered somewhat awesome and painful but it is very rare to confront a patient who jerks away from the injection or who shows any facial reaction. Those few who were observed to shy away from an injection or to cry were children, who nonetheless, were roundly chastized, cuffed and held in place for the injection. Little girls who fuss are often reminded that the treatment they are undergoing is much less painful than childbirth, so they had better learn to handle the situation. Sometimes women will behave in a joking fashion, grossly exaggerating the pain of the treatment and provoking laughter; otherwise, the typical behavior for the woman receiving an injection is to stare vaguely into space, pull her skirt down over one hip, receive the injection and leave, without comment.

The one case treated at the dispensary which was characterized by extreme manifestation of pain was that of a young miller who had amputated three fingers in his mill and came daily to have his hand dressed. Evidently in much pain, he would scream and plead for someone to save him, while other patients waiting to see the nurse would click their tongues quietly in comment, or stare fixedly in a different direction. On the other hand, a Fulbe who fell on a tree stump and gouged a large hole out of his knee came for several days to be treated. Each time, to the admiration of the observers, he sat and stared expressionlessly into the wound while the nurse poured antiseptic into it.

Courage is greatly admired by Bariba; courage among men seems to be associated with the ethic of warriors and hunters; women have fewer occasions to demonstrate their strength of character, and courage in delivery seems to be one of the few behaviors manifested by women which are admired by men. In interviewing, many men showed obvious pride in describing how their wives had been in labor without their knowledge. Although they were in the next room, they didn't realize her condition until they heard the baby cry. It seems then, that to both men and women, delivery offers a rare and dramatic opportunity for a woman to display endurance and stoicism, qualities which are highly valued in Bariba society. For men, these qualities are typically manifest in hunting (or in warfare, in the past) whereas childbirth represents the primary opportunity for women to demonstrate their courage.

The ability to adhere to the ideals regarding stoicism in the face of pain is variable, but it has been suggested, is primarily expected of adult men and women (post-puberty). It is difficult even with sophisticated equipment to undertaken comparative studies measuring degree of pain suffered but it is clear that those Bariba women observed in this study *expressed* less pain than those of other ethnic groups where such weight is not attached to denial of pain. Women in southern Benin, for example, claim that screaming helps the baby to be born and also points out to the husband how much his wife is suffering. Manifestation of pain, as indicated by such criteria as body tenseness and verbal behavior has been found in the United States to be correlated with childbirth training (Davenport-Slack and Boylan 1974:219). One study noted that childbirth training studies have for the most part found that

> Trained women behave more calmly than do nontrained women. However, these studies have often erroneously concluded that lack of overt signs of pain means that the woman is experiencing no pain. It might tentatively be concluded from the results of the present study that training provides a model for behavior during labor and delivery rather than actually decreasing the subjective experience of pain (Davenport-Slack and Boylan 1974: 220).

The same study quoted above makes reference to the significance of self-reliance, self-control and independence as factors in predicting childbirth experience (20).

Speculating on the behavior of Bariba women during labor, it seems that women do not learn any special breathing exercises comparable to Lamaze childbirth training, nor do they seem to practice meditation, reverie, trance or hypnotism. Bariba women are, however, provided with a "model of behavior" during labor and delivery. First, from childhood girls are warned of both the dangers of birth, the desirability of motherhood as a status and the necessity for self-control. The specificity of the advice increases when a girl marries and becomes pregnant. A woman experiencing her first pregancy is carefully drilled by women her own age who have already had children and by older women in what to expect and how to behave, down to details on when and how to kneel. (This description and advice procedure may be compared to the sort of "training rehearsals for labor" employed in hypnotic procedures used in relieving pain connected with childbirth, although such training is a more focused and academic training than that received by Bariba women, cf. Hilgard and Hilgard 1975.)

Although children are never present in the room where a woman is delivering, households are physically structured such that children are fully aware that something is occurring (in the case of an assisted delivery) and can hear noises, conversation, and so forth. Correspondingly, they will notice when women of the household deliver alone, and they will notice the silence of women during labor. Before her own delivery, then, a pregnant woman has had experience, if only peripheral, in evaluating the ideal behavior of a pregnant woman. In this regard, the Bariba woman is provided with more role modeling than the typical American primipara, who probably has never been in close contact with women during labor and delivery but who has attended a childbirth preparation class.

As part of childbirth preparation, experience of pain is addressed in both cultures. As Zborowski noted, "displeasure of pain is tolerated when cultural tradition calls for its acceptance" (28). In addition, anticipation of pain may allow the individual to prepare herself and respond according to the appropriate attitude of acceptance or nonacceptance (29).[29] In the case of childbirth, one would surmise that education in most cultures would include the anticipation of some discomfort. This is certainly true in the Bariba example. However, the fact of pain being expected evidently does not mean that it is accepted; one contrast between Bariba women and American women in labor revolves around this distinction between expectation and acceptance. (Note, for example, the Bariba proverb "women suffer," which applies generally to the condition of women but particularly to bearing children.) Bariba women expect pain but also expect that it must be bearable and that no recourse exists for pain alleviation, whereas American women are advised that medication can be provided and that pain can and often should be alleviated. The manifest differences between these two groups of women, then, would be related to acceptance of the bearability of pain, and the futility of the expression of pain, rather than to differences in sensitivity.

It would be interesting to conduct cross-cultural studies on the measurement of pain, should reliable technology be developed to allow such research, in order to compare pain experience as objectively as possible. In the absence of such data, I have suggested that there is a sociocultural dimension to the pain response and that appropriate behavior in response to pain in childbirth is learned. Such behavior derives from beliefs, values and expectations regarding pain in a larger cultural context. Thus the response to pain during childbirth is related both to the culturally shared meaning of birth and the degree to which pain is considered an extraordinary phenomenon, requiring special attention. In the Bariba example, stoicism, impassivity, endurance and courage in the face of physical discomfort are valued in general in Bariba society. Women are expected to cope with pain in childbirth with absence of manifest behavior, just as men are expected to respond to a hunting injury. How to manage pain in childbirth is determined by the definition of birth as a normal albeit dangerous event and by the belief that it is not appropriate to acknowledge pain from any cause. Pain during delivery is no exception.

These conclusions are supported by the scant anthropological research on pain as a cultural phenomenon. In addition to examples cited above, Jordan notes that for Maya women, pain is an "expected part of birth," so that women learn to consider pain normal and thus bearable without medication (Jordan 1978:34). A woman does not receive much sympathy if she complains; in fact, "A woman's pain and weariness are more likely to be seen as indications of progress since the baby, it is said, is born 'in the very center of the pain'" (27). Similarly, Dutch parturients, who also deliver in a non-medicating medical system, tend to manifest less pain than do American women. In Holland, because birth is defined as a natural event, women are not given drugs, although under similar conditions in the United States, they would be medicated. In contrast, Jordan comments that "American women who are attended by professional experts with an elaborate technology for alleviating pain, indeed suffer a great deal," especially given a medical setting where the woman must demonstrate to the medical personnel her need for medication (36). Moreover, in Sweden, one finds an increasingly widespread belief that pain in childbirth cannot be tolerated, and a correspondingly augmented use of medication to relieve pain (Jordan personal communication).

Given that pain has a cultural dimension, how do Bariba women manage to control the expression of their discomfort? The fact that Bariba women are advised to work as long as possible during labor, at ordinary household activities, and to walk around even when they are unable to work, seems likely to act as a diversion for the parturient similar to breathing exercises. Correspondingly, it seems possible that Bariba women, in attempts to "act" as if they were not in labor and to continue normal activities, are engaging in dissociation, a technique sometimes utilized by long-distance runners. Dissociation is a cognitive strategy which can be used for coping with pain by "thinking about something else" and deliberately cutting oneself off from the sensory feedback which would normal be received from the body (Psychology Today 4/78).

The following account of the first pregnancy of an 18-year-old Bariba schoolgirl, originally from the village of Doh, will indicate how the parturient may attempt to follow advice, her responses to labor and her strategies for coping with pain.

8.3. PREGNANCY (BY NICOLE)

I had my son involuntarily. Why is this? Because I didn't want to disappoint my husband. I was in 2ìeme (11th grade). After my menstruation, I had sexual relations with him during ten days. And after that I kept myself from going to him. But the 15th day after my period he begged me. I didn't want to give in to him because it was the day of my ovulation [she learned this in 10th grade]. But he insisted and finally I gave in to him. After this blow, I was very sure that I would become pregnant. Two weeks after I should normally have gotten my period, alas, I didn't have it; I was pregnant.

At one month of pregnancy, I already felt tired and I always wanted to sleep. I was nauseated and everything that I saw made me want to vomit. All I did was mix *acassa* [corn paste] and water, morning, noon and night. In my second month, my cousin and her husband, with whom I was living, quickly understood that I was pregnant.

Therefore my cousin told me not to drink any more *acassa* or during my delivery, I would lose too much water. I continued going to school anyway. In the fourth month, I could feel the child in my stomach. It was mango season and they [cousins] forbade me to eat mangoes. However, I hid and at lots of them. They told me mangoes make the labor hurt very much. They forbade me to sleep on my back or the umbilical cord would roll around the child; they forbade me to eat lizard (*daba*), to walk outside at night because evil spirits might change the child (into a monster) in my stomach. They advised me to work a lot so that the blood would circulate well . . . They told me to eat well because I was no longer alone. They told me not to tell anyone if I was in labor. [She went back to live at the Mission near her village.] The moment arrived, I was in labor three days and no one knew. The second night of labor I thought, what can I do to explain how I am acting? Then a scorpion bit me and I used that as an excuse. That night the nuns and my friends went to a film and I was happy because I could suffer alone.

When the nun guessed that I was in labor, she called me but the head was already coming out.

8.4. CONCLUSION

The preceding cases demonstrate the types of situations in which matrones are called to assist at deliveries, and indicate both that matrones hold in common midwifery techniques and practices and that clients and practitioners share expectations regarding appropriate and relevant diagnosis and treatment of obstetrical complications (e.g., fumigation for *tigpiru*, breech indicating witchcraft, "washing" medicines to accelerate labor.) One might argue, then, that patients and practitioners shared models of clinical reality. Kleinman et al. have argued that "Through diagnostic activities and labeling, health care providers negotiate with patients medical 'realities' that become the object of medical attention and therapeutics" (Kleinman et al. 1978a:254). I reiterate here that the degree to which models of clinical reality are shared strongly influences clients' choices of service or practitioner. Thus selection of birth assistance by Bariba women is affected by assumptions shared with matrones regarding the practice of midwifery.

The patient-practitioner encounters described above also provide information on the decision-making process in obstetrical crises. In all the cases discussed in this section, the initial impetus for requesting birth assistance came from the onset of a complication of pregnancy or labor. In one case (that of Sako), those observing initially were not aware of a complication but in retrospect, it became clear that the parturient was fearful for reasons of her own. Her labor did turn out to be complicated – this was blamed on the woman herself by everyone except me, who blamed the delayed labor on her height. Overall, however, the major factor leading to a decision to seek help was the presence of a complication or abnormality. Thus Adama feared a premature baby was a witch who would harm her during labor; Sako was referred to the nurse by a matrone who diagnosed a problem – a "high" baby, and overlong pushing plus a perplexing attitude on the part of the parturient; Ganigi experienced a prolapsed cord, diagnosed as a folk illness. The appropriate specialist was consulted and when she failed, my advice was asked. My advice being unacceptable, a second matrone was consulted. When she met no success, my advice was acted upon (reminiscent of Janzen's argument that alternative decisions may be offered within the decision-making group; if the first priority decision is found to be flawed, a lesser priority decision may subsequently be acted upon.)

In the case of breech birth, the matrone Sika was asked to attend a long labor which terminated in a clear abnormality of a buttocks presentation, and in the case of Bona, she was warned of the possibility of twins, which alarmed her. She first consulted the nurse; in his absence she called for both a matrone (selected by her elder sister) and me (her friend). She then alternated in relying on me and the matrone; when she despaired of the matrone's prowess, she asked me for medicine but switched back to the matrone at the advice of her mother-in-law. When it was determined by her husband's female relatives that her post-partum bleeding was dangerous, the nurse's apprentice, who gave injections, was consulted. (I was calling at the household regularly during that period, and offering advice, both solicited and unsolicited.)

During the collection of case material, it was often difficult to discern who was making the decisions. This difficulty was in part due to the pace at which obstetrical emergencies can occur and require action, and subsequent problems in discussing the delivery retrospectively and trying to obtain responses regarding attributions of responsibility for decisions or actions. In all cases considered here, decisions were made by women; men were kept informed of events as they arose in two cases – that of Sako, whose husband actively sought reports, and in that of Bona, which occurred on a holiday when the men were all sitting around inside the house. Men remained relatively silent and tangential to the action, however, and this was true of all cases which came to my attention, with few exceptions. These included the case where the Village Delegate's sister-in-law hemorrhaged to death and he decided to call me, after his wife tried to help her, and in some cases where male healers were consulted for severe complications. (Women of the household could consult these healers, however.) In cases at which the nurse of Pehunko assisted, he claimed that the husband was usually a trader and also a friend/acquaintance of the nurse. There were always complications in these cases too and presumably the women had first tried to deal with the situation, and then consulted the husband or head of household. It is also possible that women were reluctant to contact the male nurse (sometimes at night) in these situations.

In two cases, the decision-makers were clear; in the case of Bona, she and her elder sister decided on the nurse, and the sister on the matrone; throughout the delivery, the mother-in-law and father's brother's wife made authoritative statements which were quickly obeyed, but the elder sister was the primary assistant. At the onset of labor, the parturient gave her opinion much more than later, but she retained a voice in the proceedings throughout. In the Case of the Prolapsed Cord, the parturient's mother discussed alternatives with the parturient, me, and the second matrone and seemed to make the final decision herself. The parturient acquiesced tearfully, but the tears were attributed by others to fear, not to disagreement with the decision. The last case presented, that of Nicole, the student who tried to deliver alone but was discovered at the end of the second stage of labor by the nun, expresses the prototype of the Bariba woman attempting to conform to ideal behavior during labor and delivery.

Generally, the conclusion set forth in the Case of Bona seems applicable over a wider spectrum of cases. That is, patients and their relatives utilized indigenous and cosmopolitan health personnel and medicines both alternatively and consecutively, although in this set of cases, priority was mainly for the assistance of a matrone first. However, even when the parturient was treated in the dispensary, relatives and matrones maintained an active interest and often a treatment role in the case. Success in treatment was then attributed to the person who had intervened within the time period closest to the outcome of the delivery. This pragmatic approach to obstetrical care in national health facilities should be qualified by the note that in larger clinics or in administrative centers such as Kouande, personnel do not usually allow mixed treatments. This approach seems restricted to home deliveries and smaller, more informal dispensaries or clinics.

CHAPTER 9

UTILIZATION OF NATIONAL HEALTH SERVICES FOR MATERNITY CARE IN THE DISTRICT OF KOUANDE

Whereas preceding discussion has focused primarily on home deliveries, this chapter will provide a consideration of the factors influencing women to select a national health service delivery rather than a home delivery. Social characteristics of patients and health service utilization patterns will be examined in the context of the Pehunko dispensary and the 32-bed maternity clinic of Kouande. In addition I will compare mortality and morbidity in home deliveries and clinic deliveries and consider related implications for selection of birth assistance.

9.1. CLINIC vs HOME DELIVERY: A PEHUNKO SAMPLE

Of 117 women of reproductive age interviewed who represent approximately 43% of the estimated population of women of reproductive age in Pehunko, 95 women, or 81% delivered all their children (ever born) at home. Of the remaining women, 9% delivered all their children at a maternity clinic; 8% delivered the first child at a maternity clinic but subsequent children in home deliveries, and 3% delivered first children in home deliveries and subsequent children at maternity clinics. The majority of those women who delivered all their children in maternity clinics might be categorized as wives of upwardly mobile men, primarily wives of civil servants and traders.

9.2. UTILIZATION OF THE PEHUNKO DISPENSARY

Records exist for 43 deliveries supervised at the Pehunko dispensary in 1975–76. No records were kept during 1976–77, although nurse's aides estimated that the nurse assigned to Pehunko at that time attended approximately 13 deliveries. One possible explanation for the diminished number of cases is that the nurse serving the village during that period became particularly noted for skill in deliveries, whereas the nurse serving in 1976–77 was fundamentally a nurse for endemic diseases who assisted at deliveries because no one else was available. In this regard, the significance of the personality and reputation of the nurse should be noted as an influence on selection of medical assistance. A case in point is a former male nurse in Pehunko, who was extremely inaccessible to the population and was known to cheat patients financially. Eventually he lost almost all his clientele and was transferred out by the Ministry of Health.

A consideration of the social characteristics of the women who chose to deliver at the dispensary during 1976 shows that all 43 were under age 30. The occupations of the husbands of the women varied, as is shown in Table 14.

TABLE 14
Occupations of husbands of women delivering at Pehunko dispensary in 1976

Occupation	Percentage
Agriculture	44
Commerce	21
Civil service	9
Other (mechanic, carpenter, mason, chauffeur, photographer)	26

It is difficult to assess the significance of these percentages because data on the distribution of occupations in the general population are lacking, or if available, are not reliable.

In the agglomeration of Pehunko center and its neighborhoods (population 2,000), farmers represent over 90% of the population; civil servants 0.8% of the population; and traders with shops approximately 0.4% of the population. From the information available, it appears that wives of farmers are less likely to deliver at the dispensary than one would expect from their distribution in the village population. Contrastingly, wives of traders, civil servants and miscellaneous professions are more highly represented than their numbers in the population at large.

Additional information exists for January and February, 1977. During this period, seven women delivered at the dispensary. Five of the women had attended prenatal consultations held in Pehunko by Professor Alihonou of the National School of Midwifery in December, 1976. These women claimed that they had been told at the consultations that they should deliver at the dispensary. Three of the women experienced difficulties and all had lengthy labors at home (8 to 12 hours) before coming to the dispensary. At least one had been assisted by a matrone until the matrone admitted her capabilities had been exhausted.

With regard to the occupational status of the husbands of these parturients, five of the seven were traders, one was a nurse's aide, and one a mason. Again, traders and other non-agricultural occupations are over-represented in comparison to their proportion in the population. Observation of cliques of women in Pehunko suggests that gossip networks among families engaged in the same occupation probably stimulated some of the women to deliver at the dispensary; in addition the well-publicized prenatal consultations probably had an effect since some women did cite the consultation as a reason for selecting the dispensary.

Of these 1977 deliveries, only one was a primipara. Correspondingly, of the 43 deliveries in 1975–76, five were primiparas (12%). Thus it does not seem that women are any more likely to come to the dispensary for a first birth than for subsequent births.

Additionally, I observed several deliveries in 1977 which were not recorded in dispensary dossiers. These included a civil servant's wife who was a friend of the nurse's aide; a woman referred by a matrone after several hours of "pushing" at home; a woman in labor for 12 hours at home; and the daughter of a woman who had recently delivered a stillborn child. Another woman arrived at the dispensary in labor but the nurse was out-of-town. This woman had been warned to expect twins and was fearful of delivering alone. The death of a woman who delivered alone at home and suffered a post-partum hemmorhage in June, 1977 provoked a number of prenatal consultations and discussion among women of the benefits of delivering at the dispensary but it is too soon to evaluate the effects of that misfortune.

For whatever reason women select the dispensary, most expect immediate action and results. At four deliveries observed in 1977, after several hours at the dispensary, families became anxious and supplied the parturient with indigenous medicines (for massage and by mouth) to supplement such injections as the nurse might have administered. On two occasions, an indigenous midwife was called in to evaluate the situation and in one case where a woman spent three days in labor, two matrones were called, consecutively. This intermingling of indigenous and cosmopolitan medicine may be related to uncertainty about the power of "modern medicine," but is also related to the belief that if a medicine is appropriate for the problem it will take effect quickly (within 15 to 30 minutes for delivery medicines). Correspondingly, in the traditional medical system, most healers possess a small number of medicines, or sometimes only one, designed to treat a particular condition. In the event of failure, the healer advises the client to try elsewhere. Bariba behavior at the dispensary, then, conforms to indigenous practice in seeking medical relief.

9.2.1. *Summary Points*

The above consideration of deliveries at the Pehunko dispensary from 1975–1977 suggests the following conclusion:

(1) Primiparas are no more likely to deliver at the dispensary than multiparas.

(2) Women are likely to arrive more than two hours prior to delivery but are not likely to arrive at the onset of labor.

(3) Husbands are likely to be engaged in commerce, civil service, or other non-agricultural occupations; cultivators' wives are numerous but under-represented in proportion to their distribution in the total population.

(4) Gossip networks may be stimulating some women to deliver at the dispensary. This gossip pertains both to "neutral" news that a friend or neighbor delivered at the dispensary, and "loaded" reports of a crisis such as maternal or infant mortality.

(5) Clients combine indigenous and cosmopolitan medicine to ensure that all possible alternatives are covered and optimal care received by the parturient.

9.3. PEHUNKO WOMEN AT THE KOUANDE MATERNITY CLINIC

During 1976, thirty-one women from Pehunko delivered at the Kouande maternity clinic. Of these cases, five were probably evacuated from Pehunko for complications (inferred from maternity clinic records); three others delivered at home and came to the maternity clinic afterwards. Given that Pehunko is located 37 kilometers from Kouande and transportation between the two localities is undependable, it seems most likely that the three women had gone to stay with family in Kouande during pregnancy. This practice is common for first and second births. Others may have gone to stay with family in Kouande in order to be close to the clinic, but few are likely to have left Pehunko at the onset of labor in order to deliver in Kouande.

The only other information available on Pehunko women is the occupations of husbands of the parturients. This is shown in Table 15.

TABLE 15
Occupations of husbands of Pehunko parturients

Occupation	Number	Percentage
Cultivator/herder	11	26
of which 5 probably evacuations		
Civil Servant	8	26
Trader	3	10
Tailor	3	10
Pastor	2	7
Soldier	1	3
Veteran	1	3
Mason	1	3
Laborer	1	3

Those engaged in agriculture and the civil service, then, are the most heavily represented occupational groups. In comparison with the Pehunko dispensary deliveries, however, wives of traders are much less numerous. As in Pehunko, those engaged in agriculture are less numerous than their proportion in the population would warrant, especially if one considers that of the eleven cultivators' wives who delivered in Kouande, five were cases with complications. Therefore probably less than 20% of the cases in 1976 were wives of cultivators or herders who selected the maternity for delivery without the provocation of a crisis.

9.3.1. *Summary Points*

A consideration of clinic deliveries of Pehunko women, both in the Pehunko village dispensary and at the Kouande maternity clinic suggests that village women, other than wives of upwardly mobile men such as civil servants, prefer traditional birth attendants, when assistance is sought. More precisely, wives of traders, followed in numerical importance by wives of men engaged in non-agricultural occupations, other than civil service, show a greater likelihood of choosing to deliver in a clinic than expected. In addition, wives of cultivators comprise a relatively high percentage of those delivering in clinics (44% in Pehunko, 36% of Pehunko women in Kouande). However, given that 90% of the population is engaged in agriculture, it is evident that cultivator's wives are not represented among clinic utilizers in proportion to their representation in the population at large.

9.4. THE KOUANDE MATERNITY CLINIC: GENERAL UTILIZATION

Records from the clinic dating from 1970–76 were examined in order to provide information concerning the characteristics of women delivering at the clinic during those years. Unfortunately, population statistics for the District of Kouande are scant and consequently, it was only possible to roughly estimate the expected number of births in either the village of Kouande, where the maternity clinic is located, or in the District, for comparison with the number of clinic deliveries (see note 3). I estimated that perhaps 25–30% of the district deliveries occur in the clinic but because population data are so unreliable, this estimate is not dependable. Additionally, it was possible to compile the absolute number of deliveries for each of the six years and the total from between 1970 and 1976 and to compute the distance traveled by the client between the village of residence of the patient and the clinic. This was intended to determine the significance of distance as a factor influencing use of the maternity.[30]

9.4.1. *Distance*

Of the 1,554 cases handled at the maternity, 1,226 were residents of Kouande center (see Table 16). The next most frequent sites of origin were Gbeke (6 kilometers), Orou-Kayo (9 kilometers), Sekeguru (9 kilometers), Pehunko (37 kilometers) and Guilmaro (29 kilometers). Many of the Guilmaro deliveries were evacuations of Fulbe women. According to a clinic midwife, the Fulbe women tend to be malnourished and this debilitation is associated with complications during labor and delivery. Pehunko cases have already been described as consisting mainly of women who were staying with family in Kouande or evacuations. Gbeke, Orou-Kayo and Sekeguru are relatively close to Kouande and are on well-traveled roads. The fact of location on these roads may mean both that there is more communication regarding use of the clinic and that access to a motorbike or car heading towards Kouande is facilitated. In Gbeke, for example, there is a French priest with a car who frequently travels to Kouande and will chauffeur emergency cases. Other villages closer to Kouande have sent fewer women to the clinic; this may be due to more remote locations (linked by footpaths) or greater isolation from urban influences. In this instance, Kouande center seems to serve as a generative influence, wherein residents have become habituated to using the maternity clinic, and remote villages are stimulated to

TABLE 16
Village of residence-maternity

Village	Distance	1970	1971	1972	1973	1974	1975	1976	Total
Kouande	0	159	147	142	192	203	164	199	1,226
Kataban (Katalo)	1.5	1	0	0	2	1	0	0	4
Mare	2	1	0	0	0	0	0	0	1
Bore	5	0	2	0	0	1	0	3	6
Gbeke	6	1	1	2	1	5	8	4	22
Birbukaban	7	0	0	0	0	0	0	1	1
Kpessuru (Gassunonga)	8	2	0	3	0	0	1	3	9
Fo	9	0	0	1	1	0	1	0	3
Gnikene	9	0	0	0	1	0	0	0	1
Orou-Kayo	9	5	4	7	11	4	4	8	43
Sekeguru	9	1	4	4	6	8	5	2	30
Tokoro	9	0	0	0	0	0	0	1	1
Tanse	10	0	1	0	0	0	0	3	4
Kpessera	11	0	0	0	1	0	0	0	1
Ganikperu (Ganiha)	12	0	2	0	5	2	1	0	10
Kabare (Danni)	14	0	0	1	1	0	0	0	2
Gnekenebanssou	15	0	0	1	2	3	2	1	9
Kilibo	15	0	0	0	0	1	0	0	1
Makru	16	2	0	0	1	1	1	0	5
Tiku	16	0	0	1	0	1	0	0	2
Niaissera	17	3	0	0	2	0	1	1	7
Niarusu	17	0	1	0	2	0	2	0	5
Niaro (Ketere)	18	2	1	0	3	1	2	0	9
Maka	18	0	1	0	0	0	1	0	2
Kouba	21	2	1	0	1	0	1	0	5
Koko	26	0	1	0	0	0	0	0	1
Pouya	26	0	0	0	0	0	1	0	1
Yareku	28	0	1	0	0	0	0	0	1
Guilmaro	29	1	5	1	0	3	2	1	13
Pehunko	37	4	7	6	3	6	7	3	36
Kpaku	43	0	0	0	0	0	0	1	1
Gbweru	46	0	0	0	1	0	0	0	1
Sayakru	49	0	0	0	0	0	0	0	0
Tobre	51	1	0	0	1	3	0	0	5
Yemasson	59	0	0	0	1	0	0	1	2
Nassoukou	62	1	0	0	0	1	0	0	2
Unspecified		1	6	2	0	2	2	4	17
Unreasonable*		9	15	13	5	5	13	5	65
Total		196	200	184	243	251	239	241	1,554

* Residence cited probably that of husband; woman living in Kouande.

use clinic services through gossip networks such as information passed on market days when residents of neighboring villages are drawn to Kouande. On the other hand, when some more distant villages show greater representation, this may be due to the presence of civil servants, particularly agricultural agents, located in those villages, or to evacuations.

9.4.2. *Prenatal Consultations*

Many more women come to prenatal consultations than deliver at the clinic. Moreover, women from outlying villages who come regularly to consultations are not likely to deliver at the maternity clinic. The clinic system is for Kouande center consultations to be held on Tuesdays and for village women to come on Fridays. Most of the women who attend Friday consultations do not deliver at the clinic. The reason for this seems to be primarily one of distance, together with the problem of not knowing when labor will begin and not considering starting for the clinic until after the onset of labor.

TABLE 17
Prenatal consultations and clinic deliveries

Year	Total consulted	Total delivered
1976	95	18
1977 (1–6/77)	31	9

TABLE 18
Consultations by residence

Year	Kouande	Outlying villages	Unknown
1976	48	46	1
1977 (1–6/77)	15	16	–

TABLE 19
Deliveries of consultees by residence

Year	Kouande	Outlying villages
1976	16	2
1977 (1–6/77)	9	0

Even Kouande women often arrive at the clinic when delivery is imminent. Others deliver en route or at home. In the latter cases, the baby is brought to the maternity, still attached to the placenta, for the midwife to cut the cord and clean the baby.

TABLE 20
Home and en route deliveries by year

	1970	1971	1972	1973	1974	1975	1976
Number	23	14	16	35	40	50	23
Percentage of total	12	7	9	14	16	21	10

The high percentage of home and en route deliveries in 1973, 1974 and 1975 provoked the midwife to announce late in 1976 that women should cease bringing "basin babies" to the maternity and that mothers should refrain from "going to the woods to get kindling" during the ninth month of pregnancy. The latter statement was in response to the claim that the women couldn't make it to the clinic because they were far from home, collecting wood, at the onset of labor.

Probably reasons for these home and en route deliveries include:

(1) Distance of clinic from site of residence.
(2) Attitudes towards waiting at the maternity during labor – women claimed, in informal discussion, that if a woman waits at the clinic, she is forced to walk around, lie on the table, and is looked at. Modesty is often offered as an explanation for having arrived at the clinic when delivery was imminent. With reference to the Bariba particularly, this corresponds to the traditional ideal that a woman should hide the fact that she is in labor as long as possible; she should continue working as long as she is able and if others suspect she is in labor, they should pretend to be unaware. Thus because of their reluctance to arrive overly early at the clinic, some women deliver on the road or never leave home.

9.4.3. *Reasons for Utilizing the Clinic*

During the months of May, June and July 1977, 33 women who delivered at the maternity clinic were interviewed regarding their reasons for delivering at the clinic rather than at home. The most frequent responses were:

(1) So the midwife can save me if I suffer.
(2) At prenatal consultations, the midwife told us all to deliver at the clinic.

The complete breakdown of responses is shown in Table 21.

TABLE 21
Responses given for clinic utilization

Response	Number	Percentage
Save us if we suffer	10	30
Advised at consultation	7	21
My friends come	4	12
To assure birth certificate	4	12
Had a difficult delivery	2	6
Delivered on road, was brought	2	6
Husband is a civil servant	1	3
No response	3	9

Civil servants' wives in Pehunko also gave as a reason for preferring to deliver at the clinic the fact that their husbands were civil servants, a characteristic which is relevant from two perspectives. One is that civil servants are among those most familiar with bureaucracy and the mechanics of the family allocation system, which particularly pertains to civil servants. This system operates so that a parent presents a child's birth certificate at the local government office, fills in certain forms and receives a trimonthly supplement for the child until the child reaches age 18, or longer if the child is in school. In order to acquire a birth certificate without delivering at the clinic, the parent must pay a 1,000 franc fine; thus a person familiar with the procedure for receiving family allocations would encourage his wife to deliver at the maternity. In addition, delivery at a maternity clinic is associated with "urbanism" so that civil servants transferred from large towns to villages may send their wives to the clinic to emphasize the differences between their educated urban background and the local milieu.

Although the 33 women described in this section are only a small fraction of maternity patients, it is interesting to note that over 70% of interviewed women who had delivered during May, June and July, had delivered all their children at a maternity. Apparently, then, most of the women interviewed consistently chose the same type of birth assistance.

Contrastingly, women interviewed in Pehunko who had one or more deliveries at the clinic but others at home have as reasons for not continuing to patronize the clinic: transportation problems; cost (especially transport); home responsibilities (no one to leave the children with, no one to cook for husband); no relatives in Kouande (no one to bring food to clinic, or wash the baby). In some clinics in southern Benin, women have formed the habit of arriving at the clinic well in advance of the expected onset of labor and living at the clinic until delivery, according to a government midwife. This approach would alleviate the problem of finding locomotion at the last minute, but the other inhibiting factors remain.

The most difficult factor to evaluate is the significance of values such as courage, modesty, or fear of "abnormal" (witch) children in evoking hesitation to use a modern clinic. To give one example, displaying one's genitals, as is required at the clinic, is a breach of modesty. Another frequently expressed concern is that if a woman delivers in the lithotomy position, the child will rise back up into the uterus rather than descend and be delivered. Some women also claim they cannot push efficiently while lying down.

The value of courage among the Bariba was referred to earlier. To recapitulate, a woman demonstrates her courage by delivering alone and not calling for assistance until her child is delivered. Requiring assistance for an uncomplicated birth is considered shameful. In addition, women fear that government midwives will not report to the mother the position of the child at delivery. This is alarming because a breech birth signifies a witch child, against whom precautions should be taken. Flexibility of options in responding to a witch child (e.g., infanticide) may be reduced by a clinic delivery. Such factors tend to constrain women from selecting the maternity clinic as a therapeutic alternative.

In considering clinic utilization in contrast to the preferred birth practices of the majority of the population, the factors of central importance might be categorized as (1) role modeling and (2) boundary maintenance behavior. The significance of role modeling derives from the fact that initially, the core of the clientele of the Kouande Maternity Clinic was drawn from among southern civil servants who had been transferred north. These civil servants came from southern urban areas, were educated, and had experience with cosmopolitan medical care which has longer history and is both more accessible and more heavily utilized in the south than in the north. In addition to this category of clinic clients, employees of Catholic and Protestant missionaries were encouraged by their employers to utilize the clinic. It seems, then, that this original clinic clientele served as a source of new information and an example of innovative behavior to populations in the Kouande locale.

Moreover, reports of successful obstetrical interventions in cases given up by local matrones and transferred to the clinic (sometimes at the urging of expatriates such as priests, nuns, or agricultural advisors) provided an alternative perspective to prospective clients who viewed clinic utilization as incomprehensible behavior. Thus as Barth has suggested, people's allocations of time and resources are determined by " . . . the pay-offs that they hope to obtain and their most adequate bases for predicting these pay-offs are found in their previous experience or in that of others in their community" (Barth 1967:668). People may make mistakes in evaluation but learn as they judge outcomes of alternatives, through experience. Correspondingly, Bariba acquired and continue to acquire new information and new bases for assessing the function, benefits, and detriments of clinic deliveries from a core of clinic patrons, originally "foreigners," who served as role models.

A second factor cited as significant in explaining clinic utilization was boundary maintenance behavior. Civil servants' wives, when questioned as to why they delivered in a clinic rather than at home invariably responded flatly that "civil servants use clinics; we don't have babies at home." To civil servants, especially southerners from an urban background who have been transferred to positions in the rural north, utilization of national health services ("modern medicine") differentiates the educated urban elite from the uneducated rural population (cf. Hanks 1963; Foster 1973; Eramus 1977).

Similarly, civil servants have historically been identified by northerners as foreigners and further, as members of the elite, linked with the national government. Institutions such as the maternity clinic were equally associated with the national government, southerners, and the elite. Thus rural Bariba (as well as members of other ethnic groups in the region) have maintained the distinction between "Bariba" and foreigners by *not* patronizing the clinic. However, the increasing presence of the national government in the Bariba region in aspects of life such as cultivation, marketing, ideological orientation, enforcement of compulsory education requirements, immunization campaigns and military training seems to portend a blurring of the boundaries between Bariba and non-Bariba and northerners versus southerners. It seems also that Bariba with aspirations to upward mobility, such as wealthy traders, are adopting patterns of "civil servant" behavior as a means of redefining their status and attempting to enhance their prestige. One might argue, then, that increasing clinic utilization by traders and peasants is a precursor to the breakdown of boundary maintenance behavior and represents a facet of the process of national integration.

9.4.4. *Features of the Model*

Reviewing the goals of Bariba women at delivery, one finds that the goals of a farmer's wife in Pehunko and a trader's wife in Kouande might be defined as follows:

Farmer's Wife	Trader's Wife
live mother and baby	live mother and baby
witchcraft control	aspirations to upward mobility
manifestations of high standards of female behavior	prestige associated with 'civil servant' behavior
minimization of infrastructural costs	minimization of infrastructural costs

Selection of birth assistance and utilization of a type of health service derive from attempts to achieve the above sets of goals as fully as possible.

Thus far a set of factors has been shown to influence women's obstetrical care choices. These factors might be conceptualized as monetary and non-monetary constraints and incentives, which might be diagramatically represented as is shown in Figure 4. Either monetary or non-monetary costs may act as the determining factors in obstetrical care decision-making (Riley and Sermsri 1974:58). However, it is important to emphasize the critical effect of monetary costs, and constraints related to the health infrastructure, such as transportation, fees, support services for maternity patients, and home obligations. Thus a woman who is considering delivery in the Kouande clinic must have transportation at the appropriate time, money to pay for the transport, relatives nearby to feed her while she is staying at the clinic, and someone to undertake home responsibilities during her absence. In many cases, such factors may render the utilization of the clinic *not a real option.*

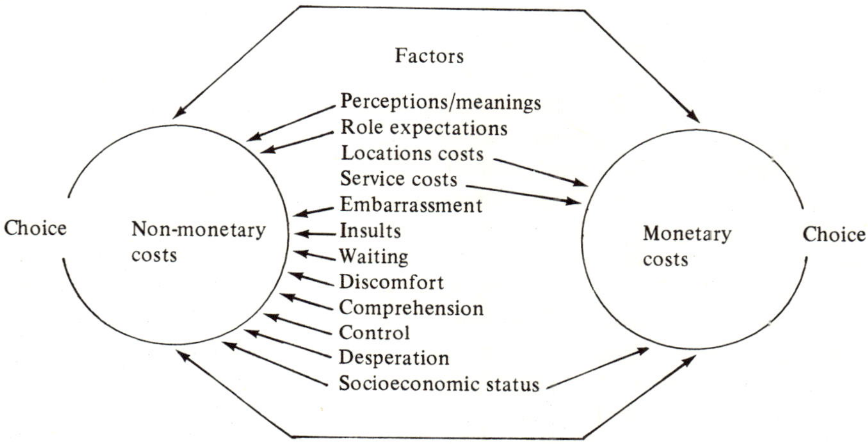

Fig. 4. Monetary and non-monetary cost factors affecting choice.

One must also ask, if no structural factors or monetary costs inhibited utilization, or if the infrastructure facilitated utilization, would women exploit maternity services? The answer evident in this discussion is that many would not, in part due to a variety of conflicting values which may be called into consideration in selecting birth assistance. Among these are modesty, courage, competence credibility, familiarity and prestige aspirations. Which values will dominate may depend on the situation. For example, the husband's status may outweigh the wife's desire for privacy. Depending on the sanctions the woman may fear if she disregards her husband's preferences, his may be the deciding influence. Contrastingly, even in the event that her husband desires a maternity delivery, if the woman has returned to stay with her own family, the option of her relatives, particularly elderly women, may be decisive.

The data suggest that at least three types of factors operate in the selection of birth assistance. These include:

(1) social infrastructural factors;
(2) personal costs;
(3) values and other non-monetary costs.

This set of factors was found to interact to faciliate or inhibit choice of a maternity care option. Thus:

NO CHOICE	⟷	Social infrastructure personal cost	⟷	CHOICE
		↕		
OPTION REFUSAL	⟷	Non-monetary costs (Values)	⟷	OPTION

Unfortunately, the data do not offer sufficient evidence to enable weighing these factors, except in indicating extremes. The factors should not be regarded with a higher degree of specificity than is warranted by people's decision-making process, in which the outcome is rarely due to a discrete element. One can say, though, that any factor may prohibit utilization and negate the possibility of a real choice. Moreover, where all factors operate together, whether to facilitate or inhibit utilization, the odds are that the decision is predictable. Thus a woman with little cash income available, living in Guilmaro (29 kilometers journey from Kouande, no regular transport) who has always delivered alone, is very unlikely to choose the maternity clinic except in the event of an emergency evacuation, whereas a rich trader's wife or wife of a civil servant living one kilometer from the clinic is most likely to do so.

In the intermediate range, where there appears to be no cluster of high monetary costs, nor relative absence of such costs, it is difficult to predict choices. The problem which arises seems to be that as the comparative differences in benefits and costs narrows between alternatives, it becomes progressively more difficult to predict which choice will be preferred; thus where there seems to be little to recommend one choice over another, individuals may seem to be choosing at random, by whimsy, or due to the greater visibility of one alternative at a critical moment. It may, then, be inherently impossible to predict behavior in this middle range.

9.4.5. *Morbidity and Mortality*

A question which arises in examining the utilization of medical facilities such as dispensaries and clinics is the following: are people making rational decisions in deciding to use or not use a national health facility for obstetrical services. "Rationality," as defined in chapter 1, refers to choosing the most effective means to reach a goal (or most preferred goal when a set of goals is involved), however that goal is defined. A consideration of Bariba birth has indicated that Bariba hope to achieve multiple goals at delivery and primary among these goals are "live mother" and "live baby." In discussing the utilization of national health services for maternity care, then, one must consider to what extent dispensaries and clinics represent the most effective means to reaching the goal of "live mother and baby."

Various writers have suggested that choice of a health service or form of therapy is based on previous evidence obtained by the client population regarding the efficacy of the alternatives available (Colson 1971:227). Other observers referring to obstetrical care in particular have commented that obstetrical services tend to attract clients more quickly than other services, due to the observed benefits of improved care (Maclean 1976, Foster 1962, Landy 1977).

The subsequent section will address the above issues from both an emic and an etic perspective.[31] First, from an ethic perspective, what does available information regarding morbidity and mortality in home deliveries and in national health services suggest with respect to the quality of care available in those settings and correspondingly, what are the implications of this quality of care for service utilization. Second, from an emic perspective, how do local populations assess the quality of care in national health services with respect to the delivery goal of "live mother and baby" and finally, to what extent do the Bariba data support the suggestion of other writers that prospective clients select a health service on the basis of "observed frequencies of successful outcomes" (Erasmus 1957).

9.4.6. *The Etic Perspective*

Government policy, which increasingly advocates maternity deliveries and decries traditional practices, assumes that people are irrational or not maximizing the potential for effective health care if they do not choose to employ the available resources. This policy position is not, however, based on an assessment of morbidity and mortality statistics in health services throughout the country.

Because of the absence of birth and death registrations, it is difficult to estimate mortality rates. Information on maternal mortality proved impossible to obtain on a systematic basis due to the prevalent Bariba attitudes toward maternal deaths. Although some attempt was made at interviewing matrones regarding maternal deaths which they had encountered or remembered, this questioning was dropped due to distaste and outright refusal to answer the question among all the matrones.

Information on maternal mortality was therefore acquired by hearsay. Obtaining such information was facilitated by the custom of requiring pregnant women and women carrying babies on their backs to flee the village (or neighborhood, in the case of a large village) until the parturient was buried. News of such an event was noteworthy; in addition, the Pehunko nurse, during journeys to outlying villages for treatment of endemic diseases, often learned of unusual occurrences such as maternal death. By this somewhat haphazard but reasonably accurate method, it can be stated that at least three maternal deaths occurred among women residing in a population area for which I estimate 272 women of reproductive age during the period of data collection of twelve months. Accounting for child spacing practices, one might expect from 21 to 30 deaths per 1,000 live births. This variance is related to alternative census data on the Pehunko regions, as follows: (computed with the assistance of the staff of the University of California Maternal and Child Health Project in Cotonou, R. P. Benin).

Option (1). Based on personal census of the Pehunko agglomeration.

if there are 272 women of reproductive age
10% infertile
= 245 women

if each woman delivers every 29 months, 101 births would be expected annually for this population. Three maternal deaths per 101 births can be extrapolated to 30 deaths per 1,000 births.

Option (2). If the population as officially listed is used as a base, there would be 375 women of reproductive age, which following the same computation, would suggest an expected 140 births annually and a maternal mortality rate of 21 per 1,000 births.

The maternal mortality rate, then, seems to be between 21 and 30 per 1,000. If, however, the pregnancy interval is less than my estimation, the number of expected births would be greater and the mortality rate lower; also, with such small numbers, an annual change of one death would greatly alter the mortality rate – thus two deaths in 101 births would result in a mortality rate of 20 per 1,000 and two deaths in 140 births in a mortality rate of 14 per 1,000.

In comparison to the range of 21 to 30 deaths per 1,000 in 1976, the rate in the maternity clinic in the provincial capital of Natitingou in 1975 was estimated at 14. per 1,000. In comparing these maternal mortality rates, the hypothesis to be tested was that maternal mortality in the national health clinic in Natitingou differed from the mortality in the rural region of Pehunko. This hypothesis was designed in order to contrast the quality of care in the two settings as manifest by mortality statistics and to examine the possibility that government policy is incorrect in advocating use of maternity clinics based on the assumption that clients are likely to experience more successful delivery outcomes in a maternity setting than with home delivery. Correspondingly, comparison of mortality rates was expected to assist in interpreting Bariba assessments of the benefits to be gained from utilizing a maternity service.

If the mortality rate of 21 per 1,000 is compared to the clinic rate of 14 per 1,000, the results are as follows:

	Died	Lived	Total
Observed	3	137	140
Expected	2	138	140

x^2 = 0.00361. The critical value, set at 95% confidence level, was 3.841, therefore the results were not significant.

If the mortality rate of 30 per 1,000 is compared to the clinic rate of 14 per 1,000, the results are:

	Died	Lived	Total
Observed	3	98	101
Expected	1.4	99.6	101

x^2 = 2.09. Therefore, again, the difference in the maternity figures was not significant.

It seems, then, that the hypothesis that the mortality in the Natitingou clinic differs significantly from the mortality at home in the Pehunko region is not supported In order to examine more closely the meaning of this conclusion, some additional aspects of morbidity in the rural, home-delivery setting and in clinic settings will be considered. As a preliminary to evaluating morbidity and morality in the rural area and in order to assess the kinds of complications with which a matrone might be expected to contend, prenatal consultations were conducted with a sample of 50 pregnant women in the Pehunko area. These consultations were organized and supervised by Professor Alihonou, Director of Obstetrical and Gynecological Services, National University of Benin.

Prenatal screening suggested that Bariba women enter pregnancy in generally good health. Particular attention was paid to hemoglobin levels in this sample, due to the assumption that rural women would likely suffer nutritional deficiencies leading to anemias. Resulting debilitation might cause complications in labor and delivery (cf. Knottenbelt 1973; Foster 1968; Mati and Hatimy 1971). Among the 45 women tested, the average hemoglobins were found to be 9.32 grams hemoglobin per 100 ml blood, compared to an average of 12 for a control group of 106 non-pregnant women. (These hemoglobins were measured using a hemoglobinometer and were checked by two observers.)

According to the Geigy Pharmeceutical Scientific Tables on blood values (1975) average hemoglobin levels for non-pregnant women were 13.1 grams and for pregnant women (34 weeks) 11.1, with an average drop of two grams during pregnancy. Assuming that these levels are based on hemoglobins of white women, it is useful to note the work of Garn et al. (1975) who showed a difference in black-white hemoglobin levels (where income was held constant) of 1 g/100 ml blood; the authors speculated that a genetic difference was responsible. Based on Garn's data, the mean lowest recorded hemoglobin value of pregnant black women (unsupplemented by injection) was 10.2, with a standard deviation of 1.6. Bariba women, then, are concentrated at the lower end of this distribution (Garn, personal communication, from Perinatal Collaborative Study).

Using the above figures, one might expect a non-pregnant black woman to have a hemoglobin level of 12.1 and a pregnant black woman, a level of 10.1. The Pehunko sample of non-pregnant women, then showed an average hemoglobin level of 12, comparable to the expected "normal" level for black, non-pregnant women. The pregnant women, however, showed a drop of 2.7 grams Hb (as compared to the "normal" drop of 2 grams) during pregnancy. This augmented drop may be due to lack of iron supplements during pregnancy, or hypothetically, to dietary changes, but none of the latter could be determined. Seasonal factors did not seem significant in explaining the difference; pregnant women were tested in December, at the beginning of the dry season when food supplies, including some green leaves, remained plentiful; non-pregnant women were tested in February. If a level of 10 grams Hb is considered a normal level, then 70% of the Pehunko pregnant women would be considered anemic; however, the consulting obstetrician, Alihonou, noted that in current local clinical practice, women were not considered anemic with a hemoglobin of 10. In his experience, those with hemoglobins under 9 were referred for further diagnosis and treatment. Garn's data also suggest normal hemoglobin levels to be lower than do some other studies (Ferguson et al. 1968; Mati and Hatimy 1971; Elwood 1973).

Thus the findings of this sample of Bariba women does not support the idea that complications of pregnancy, labor and delivery are likely to be related to anemia. In addition, the finding that 106 non-pregnant women of reproductive age (i.e., "between" pregnancies) showed hemoglobin levels averaging 12 grams suggests that iron supplementation during pregnancy may not be necessary to prevent anemia after a succession of pregnancies.

The prenatal examinations also provided information regarding the effects of the kneeling position preferred at delivery by Bariba women. One might question whether women who deliver in a kneeling position, without a tradition of episiotomy, do not suffer severe tearing; such tears might then become infected. Following prenatal examinations, however, Dr. Alihonou concluded that the multiparous women showed no signs of severe scarring which would indicate previous tearing. Unfortunately he was unable to complete a further study directly devoted to this issue which would have provided valuable insights into the effects of delivery position. Where tearing does occur, the usual hygienic measures, involving strict observation of post-partum vaginal washings with hot water and strong soap, might reduce the likelihood of infection; correspondingly, puerperal fever seemed to be rare – in a one year period, the nurse was called to treat one case of high fever and severe post-partum infection. This apparent low incidence of infection also seems related to the customary hygienic measures.

As a cause of mortality, obstructed delivery should be mentioned. Although statistics are not available, several cases occurred of women who died during labor, in neighboring areas. Both the district maternity clinic and the provincial maternity clinic claim to have received cases requiring a Caesarian section; (statistics were not available) only the hospital is equipped to handle surgical procedures. In Bariba practice, the only technique devised to deal with what is believed to be an obstructed labor is an episiotomy; this procedure is said to be performed, for example, when excessive scarring from clitoridectomy inhibits the birth of the child. Other than this technique, no surgical procedures are practiced; situations where the parturient cannot deliver vaginally, then, no doubt resulted in mortality in the past and often continue to do so.

Additional information on morbidity associated with home deliveries was difficult to obtain because of the impossibility of obtaining systematic data by trained medical personnel whenever a complaint arose. Some conclusions can tentatively be drawn regarding obstetrical complications, however, based on Professor Alihonou's interpretation of reports regarding deliveries observed by the researcher and described to him.

One primary topic of interest is the treatment of complications associated with delivery of the placenta. Because of Bariba beliefs regarding the dangers of a retained placenta and the expectation that the placenta should be delivered immediately following delivery of the baby, numerous procedures have been developed to accelerate delivery of the placenta. The possibility exists that the remedial measures designed to expel the placenta such as rolling the parturient's abdomen with a broom may in fact be injurious and may, for example *provoke* retention of the placenta. Given the widespread practice of broom-rolling, it is possible that this procedure, intended as therapeutic, actually provokes complications and thus affects the morbidity rate in the region. Similarly, Bariba assessments of the therapeutic effects of bleeding and lack of indigenous medicines to arrest hemorrhage may also increase morbidity and mortality in home deliveries.

In summary, a review of complications associated with home delivery suggests that (1) Bariba women are not notably anemic and correspondingly, anemia does not produce general debilitation leading to a high rate of complications of delivery; (2) that delivery position does not seem to cause complications such as scarring (other complications were not investigated); (3) that post-partum infection seems infrequent; (4) that indigenous methods of expelling the placenta may be harmful; and (5) that indigenous midwifery does not include techniques for handling either obstructed labor or pelvic disproportions, or for arresting hemorrhage. Although it is difficult to draw conclusions regarding morbidity associated with home deliveries, one can tentatively suggest that women experiencing retained placenta, obstructed labor or hemorrhage are particularly likely to receive inadequate treatment from a matrone.

9.4.7. *The Clinic Setting*

In comparison with the risks encountered by a woman who does not consult cosmopolitan medical personnel and who delivers at home, the risks to women who utilize maternity clinics are also noteworthy. Speaking of maternity clinics in Benin in general, Takpara Issifou, in his 1976 Thesis for the Doctorate of Medicine on maternal and perinatal mortality in Benin, states that the majority of the maternity clinics in Benin are competent to deal only with eutocic deliveries (11), lacking as they do, equipment and/or capable personnel. He states that "throughout the territory, at this time, one single maternity, that of Cotonou, can resolve in a satisfactory fashion, obstetrical problems . . . " (11, my translation). Because of overworked personnel and insufficient stocks of drugs and equipment, together with tardy evacuations of complicated cases from rural areas, the quality of care available in maternity clinics suffers. Takpara also signals the problem of maternity personnel who receive parturients who have never been seen at a prenatal consultation, due to (a) absence of family allocations (b) inconvenient distances to travel and (c) time-consuming daily responsibilities (13). Maternity clinics supervise from 10 to 20% of the deliveries in rural areas. A consideration of maternal mortality in three maternities indicates a wider variation in rates. These maternities are located in three major towns: Cotonou, the capital; Parakou, the northern railhead town; and Natitingou, administrative capital of the Atakora Province and clinic to which Kouande district women would be evacuated in an emergency (19–20).

TABLE 22
Maternal mortality per clinic by year

Maternity	Years	Maternal mortality per 1,000*
Cotonou	1970	3
	1975	2
Parakou	1973	6
	1974	3
Natitingou	1973	17
	1974	15
	1975	14

* The World Health Organization has suggested as a goal for the Africa Region to bring maternal mortality down to 0.04 per 1,000 in the next 25 years (20). The rate in France in 1975 was 0.26 (43). The overall maternal mortality rate for Benin is cited by Takpara as 1.7 per 1,000 based on records from 67 clinics; however this rate seems suspiciously low given the 1975 rate at the Cotonou clinic and perhaps reflects poor recordkeeping from the smaller, rural clinics. The rate of 1.7 is, nonetheless, 6.5 times as high as that in France and corresponds to the rate in France at the turn of the century.

The difference in the maternal mortality rates in Cotonou (2) and Natitingou (14) is partly explainable in terms of factors suggested by Takpara – lack of equipment and drugs, shortage of personnel and overworked personnel, and late evacuations of exhausted parturients who are more likely to die due to their debilitated condition. Due to difficulties with records, detailed information on cause of maternal death could not be obtained for Natitingou. However, Takpara provides provocative information on 95 cases of maternal deaths in the Cotonou maternity clinic, from 1970–75. Causes of death were determined to be as illustrated in Table 23.

TABLE 23
Causes of death in the Cotonou maternity clinic

Cause of Death	No. of women	Percentage
Hemorrhage	55	56
Infection	22	23
Viral hepatitis	9	10
Surgical shock	4	4
Eclampsia	3	3
Amniotic embolism	2	2

Approximately 91% of these parturients were evacuated from towns and villages up to 130 kilometers distance from Cotonou (21). As in the Natitingou situation, then, one might speculate that some of the deaths resulted from late evacuations, as in the cases of women in labor 24 to 48 hours before being transported to Cotonou.

Interestingly, the primary cause of death was found to be hemorrhages, which were also a significant cause of maternal mortality in the Pehunko region. Infections, as was previously mentioned, do not seem to be a significant factor in maternal morbidity or mortality in the Pehunko area, and the other causes of death cited for Cotonou are also unknown or undiagnosed in rural areas. Interviewing in the Pehunko population on symptoms of eclampsia elicited no recognition; surgical shock is no doubt a factor in Natitingou, but of course not in rural areas, and hepatitis and embolisms could not be investigated because the researcher lacked the medical training to diagnose these conditions.

Looking more closely at hemorrhage as a cause of death in Cotonou, one finds hemorrhages linked to cases of uterine rupture (49%), placental delivery (26%), placenta previa (13%), premature delivery of placenta (10%) and cervical lacerations (4%). In his discussion of hemorrhage as a cause of death, Takpara makes an observation which is particularly pertinent to the data on rural Bariba women. Takpara comments that 428 women were received at the Cotonou maternity for treatment of hemorrhage associated with delivery of the placenta. Of the 428 women, 14 died. *These hemorrhages followed intemperate manoeuvers practiced on the cord or abdominal pressure immediately following delivery of the child* (23, my italics). His observation lends support to the hypothesis that the Bariba practice of rolling the abdomen with a broom immediately following delivery of the child may provoke complications and that the two deaths in the region described as due to retained placenta may more accurately be due to hemorrhage. It is also interesting that the practice of abdominal pressure is widespread among southern as well as northern ethnic groups. Cord traction is not, however, characteristic of Bariba midwifery.

In sum, one finds certain parallels in primary causes and contexts of morbidity and mortality in rural, home deliveries in the Bariba region and deliveries in the major maternity clinic in the country. Although statistics are not available, one might expect a similar correspondence between the Cotonou and Natitingou maternity clinics in causes of mortality, with the contrast that a greater percentage of patients dies in Natitingou due to factors already specified, such as shortage of supplies, personnel, and late evacuations of patients from remote rural areas.

In referring to the maternal mortality rate in Natitingou, it has already been noted that no significant difference was found between maternal mortality rates in the clinic and in the Pehunko home delivery setting. In drawing this conclusion, it is necessary to note that the factor of late evacuations leads to a situation where the Natitingou clinic serves a client population which is especially likely to die. It would be unwise, then, to lean too heavily on the conclusion that mortality does not differ in the home delivery and clinic settings, or to ignore the fact that some complications are more successfully treated at clinics, given reasonable conditions (for instance, retained placentas if the parturient has not waited unduly long before consulting at the clinic). The Kouande clinic, for example, which evacuated its worst cases to Natitingou, showed a much lower maternal mortality rate than that in Natitingou – one death in the 1970–76 period; underreporting may be at issue here, however.

In general, it seems that in cases of severe complications, the only maternity clinic in the country truly competent to provide care is located in Cotonou. Although in some circumstances local and provincial clinics in the northern region may deal successfully with problems of labor and delivery, the benefits of a clinic delivery are not always conclusively evident, based on current mortality data. Parenthetically, another issue which was not closely considered in this research was whether eutocic deliveries are more safely conducted in clinics; one authority suggested that hygienic procedures at some clinics are such that a parturient is less at risk for infection if she stays at home (Dr. C. De Sweemer, personal communication).

Finally, the question of the quality of care offered by matrones in contrast to national health services raises an issue which is much larger than that of the comparative morbidity and mortality in Pehunko home deliveries and Natitingou clinic deliveries. This issue involves a comparison between the Natitingou provincial maternity clinic and the Cotonou maternity clinic. Previously, maternal mortality rates in the two clinics were cited as 14/1,000 in 1975 and 2/1,000 in 1975 respectively – in other words, the Natitingou rate is almost seven times greater than that in Cotonou. Given the observations of Takpara and Alihonou (personal communications), it seems likely that the explanation for this differential lies largely in the budgetary priorities accorded the capital city clinic.

A brief review of the distribution of health personnel throughout the country suggests that this facet of the quality of care – availability of personnel – is directly linked to the priorities allocated to certain regions of the country. To recapitulate, the distribution of personnel in the Province de l'Atlantique (Cotonou) and in the Province de l'Atakora (Natitingou) is found in Table 24.

TABLE 24
Distribution of personnel

Personnel	Atlantique	Atakora
Doctors	15	1
Dentists	4	0
Nurses	269	90
Nurse-midwives	133	10
Total population	447,000	365,000

To give one example, if equal priority was allocated to both provinces, one would expect to find that based on the Cotonou personnel numbers, 219 nurses would be transferred to the Atakora, rather than 90; similarly, one would expect 108 nurse-midwives rather than 10.

Other information on the national budget allocations for health care is not available; however, a superficial investigation of pharmacies throughout the country will quickly indicate that north of Parakou, drugs are in scant supply and stockage is very irregular and undependable. (At the time of Alihonou's prenatal consultations in Pehunko, he was shocked to find that none of the gynecological products which he prescribed were available closer than Parakou, a distance of 177 kilometers, accessibly every five days by market truck at a cost of 2600 CFA round trip; one can also commission the driver to bring medicine which increases the cost of the product.) It is also worth remarking that in spite of the fact that the Atakora Province has the highest mortality rate in the country, health personnel are very reluctant to be transferred to this region because of the difficult working conditions, and because of the reputation of the region as a frontier outpost, characterized by xenophobia, food shortages and so forth. Thus in 1976–77, six nurses were officially transferred to the Atakora but none arrived; of ninety onsite, ten left. Clearly, the historically low priority of the Atakora in national planning, expressed here in the positioning of health personnel, which has persisted to the present, explains the extent to which facilities, resources, and personnel are available in the region. Correspondingly, the quality of care offered by national health services in the Atakora in general and in Kouande in particular is fundamentally affected by national priorities which have relegated public services in the Atakora Province to a low priority.

9.4.8. *The Emic Perspective*

Discussions with matrones and their clients indicated that certain complications are perceived as likely to be associated with pregnancy and delivery. Both matrones and women of reproductive age shared perceptions regarding morbidity associated with delivery. During interviews, matrones were questioned regarding some obstetrical complications considered common in western biomedicine. The complications discussed included: (a) fever, (b) tearing, (c) tetanus (convulsions), (d) severe bleeding, (e) breast abcess. Matrones disclaimed familiarity with all of the above, excepting breast abcess which was reported to be common and treated by cauterization. The interpretation of bleeding among Bariba women has already been discussed – bleeding is considered a healthy mechanism for cleansing the female interior of ailments. Bleeding which is excessive or is associated with death, may be interpreted as pathological but is not invariably identified as a cause of mortality. From the point of view of matrones and parturients, however, vertigo and fatigue are frequent concommitants of delivery.

In general, *tigpiru* is considered to be an extremely prevalent problem during pregnancy and delivery but is not usually considered to be life-threatening. As previously stated, Bariba believe that it is not worthwhile to seek treatment at a national health service for *tigpiru* because it is an indigenous complaint which health personnel do not know how to diagnose, nor do they have medicines to treat this complaint.

Contrastingly, in the perceptions of most women, the primary complication of delivery is a retained placenta; both matrones and their clients claim a high prevalence for this complication and comment that parturients risk death primarily from this condition. Obstructed labor is the second most dreaded complication of labor. In the event that either of these two complications should arise, matrones and women of reproductive age *do* consider the possibility of utilizing national health services.

Although women in the Kouande area have observed and been impressed with successful treatment of some obstetrical emergencies in the Kouande maternity clinic, in the perception of much of the rural population, experience has shown that women who are evacuated to a clinic because of complications of labor and delivery often die. The fact that such women may sometimes die because of delays or home treatments does not alter the end impression which equates hospitals with death. Women of Kouande, for instance, noted that women in labor sent to Natitingou for surgery die. In actuality, although accurate records could not be obtained, reports from nurse-midwives suggest that during a period of several years, a succession of women did die during Caesarian sections. Possibly this rash of deaths represented a small proportion of cases treated, but nonetheless, the effect via the rumor network of Kouande has been long-lasting.

In returning to the original question of whether women who choose not to utilize a clinic are making a rational choice, the above discussion on morbidity and mortality suggests that both in terms of the information available to them, and in light of the adequacy of the provincial health facilities as manifest by the mortality statistics, Pehunko women are selecting a reasonable alternative when they choose to stay at home to deliver. It seems incorrect to argue that women who prefer a home delivery are not safeguarding their health and that of their infants. The implication of this conclusion is that a significant change in utilization patterns, with a shift to a preference for cosmopolitan medical care, will depend in part on changes in the effectiveness of the care available.

Thus Bariba women selecting delivery assistance appear to be choosing rationally in the sense of selecting the most effective means of reaching the delivery goal of "live mother and baby." Moreover, those analysts who have suggested that client populations deciding among therapeutic options are affected by observed frequencies of successful outcomes appear to be correct in that assumption.

CHAPTER 10

CONCLUSION

10.1. IMPLICATIONS OF THE BARIBA STUDY FOR THE CROSS-CULTURAL STUDY OF MIDWIFERY

The Bariba study, by providing an in-depth examination of the comprehensive role of the indigenous midwife in a rural African society, touches on a number of concerns in cross-cultural research on obstetrics. One of the most important issues which scholars and government planners need to confront is factors influencing health care decision-making in various cultural contexts. In attempting to determine the reasons for the slow increase in the utilization of national health obstetrical services in the District of Kouande and for the continuing preference among Bariba women for maintaining indigenous birth practices, a set of salient factors emerged, which it may be useful to review.

In general, the Bariba data suggest that decisions regarding the utilization of alternative medical services are largely derived from the diagnosis of the sickness or disorder that presents a problem to the sufferer and to significant others. In the Bariba case, the possibility of witchcraft as a causative factor in complications of delivery influenced the actions of parturients, their families and birth attendants in selecting therapeutic options in that a specialist in obstetrical complications was expected to be competent to confront witchcraft in a delivery setting. Similarly, the preference for solitary delivery is associated with witchcraft beliefs. Throughout the discussion of reproduction, the status of women was assumed to be of critical significance because in Bariba society, as throughout rural Africa, reproduction is a domain of particular concern to women. In general, women's goals were presumed to be defined by their position in society and reproductive goals are one such set of goals.

The domain of reproduction represents the primary arena in which women control decision-making and carries a twofold potential for a women to enhance her prestige. First, a necessary route to achieving any position of respect and influence for a woman is to be a "mother of children," especially sons. The goal of producing many children is shared by men and women, but its achievement is largely the responsibility of women, whether via self-management of pregnancy and delivery, through communications with other women of reproductive age, or via counsel, diagnosis and treatment from elderly female specialists. Moreover, professional specialization in reproductive disorders provides one of the rare avenues for women to transcend sex as a category and to achieve fame which might surpass regional limits.

In considering women's decisions to select a type of birth setting and obstetrical assistance, it becomes evident that a Bariba woman who decides to deliver in the District Maternity Clinic is foregoing control of a customary domain of female responsibility. For example, a home delivery, whether assisted or solitary, generally remains the complete responsibility of the household women. If those who become involved choose to request assistance from a specialist, that choice is also their prerogative. If, however, a woman is contemplating a national health service delivery, she must, under most circumstances, ask permission from the male head of household. Starting with the decision to select this type of assistance, then, a woman's realm of responsibility and authority is diminished. In addition, women perceive that their control of the delivery situation is weakened in many respects – by definition, a woman who selects the maternity option cannot deliver alone and has relinquished her flexibility regarding the fate of the child; she has lost her authority to request and then accept or reject treatment offered by a matrone; and she loses the opportunity to enhance her prestige by demonstrating courage as manifest by one of the few means available to women – the solitary delivery.

Moreover, the selection of a clinic delivery removes "birth" from the context of a female specialization – in some instances a male nurse may supervise the delivery and the government nurse-midwife, although she is a female practitioner, is not perceived as occupying a role parallel to that of the Bariba matrone. Thus, although great respect is attached to the role of the matrone, this respect is not transferred to that of nurse-midwife. The nurse-midwife's functions lie outside the Bariba reproductive complex which incorporates meanings, beliefs, and practices associated with professional specialization in Bariba society, with sex roles, and with witchcraft as a causative agent of misfortune. Rather, a Bariba woman from Pehunko who delivers in the Kouande clinic is entering a domain which signifies the presence of the national government, of foreign authority, cash incomes, and bureaucratic procedures, in which midwifery is a narrow technical specialty and client and practitioner do not share concepts of the implications of reproduction.

Correspondingly, expectations held by Bariba women regarding the midwife as a particular type of practitioner were found to be significant influences affecting selection of birth assistance. Bariba women, as clients, and matrones share concepts of sickness causation and expectations regarding diagnosis, delivery goals, and midwifery techniques and practices. To her clients, the matrone is perceived as competent because she demonstrates attributes which fall within an acceptable range. Additionally, clients and matrones share expectations with respect to appropriate behavior for a parturient and regarding client-practitioner interactions.

Choice of practitioner, then, is related to role expectations held by clients regarding attributes, techniques and practices characteristic of a competent midwife. In sum, the absence of shared expectations among nurse-midwives and prospective clients regarding appropriate role behavior, differing concepts of causation of obstetrical complications and appropriate midwifery practices serve to constrain prospective clinic patients from utilizing the clinic alternative. (see Figure 5).

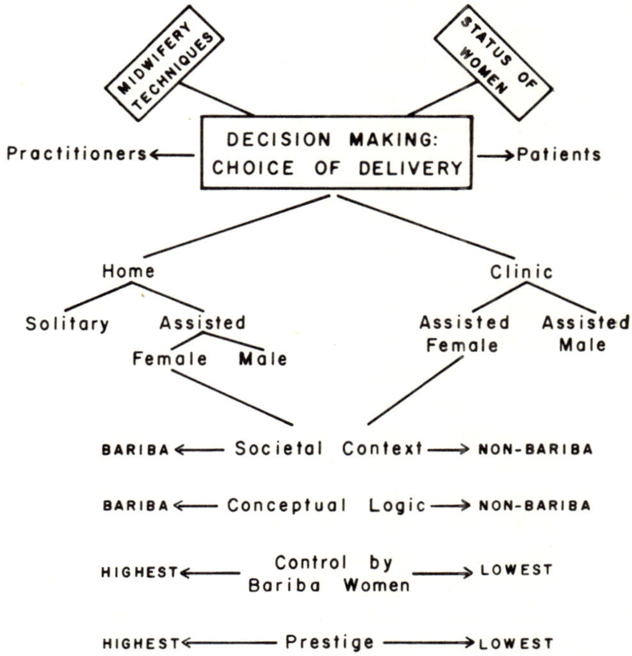

Fig. 5. Dimensions of Contrast in Obstetrical Care Choices.

Those women who use the national health maternity services tend to be women who reside within a two-kilometer radius of the clinic, who are wives of civil servants, wives of wealthy traders, and wives of men in "modern" occupations. Wives of peasants represented the lowest percentage of clinic patrons, in proportion to their representation in the population. Peasant women do, however, increasingly utilize the maternity clinic. This trend may be explained as one facet of the process of national integration, and has developed as Bariba women have acquired new information and new bases of information for assessing the function, benefits, and detriments of clinic deliveries from a core of clinic patrons, originally "foreigners," who served as role models.

10.2. THE INVOLVEMENT OF INDIGENOUS MIDWIVES IN NATIONAL HEALTH SYSTEMS

Given the constraints operating in the Bariba case, the involvement of indigenous midwives in national health systems becomes a key planning issue. A growing body of literature documents the positve and negative aspects of the utilization of indigenous healers as collaborators with cosmopolitan medical personnel,[32] and a variety of investigators have advocated some form of accomodation between indigenous and cosmopolitan medical systems (cf. Jordan 1978; Population Reports, May 1980; Good et al. 1979).[33]

Although I did not develop a detailed argument on this subject in the Bariba study, the research presented exemplifies the range and depth of data necessary to make valid judgments regarding the utility and practicality of training indigenous midwives. In addition, it attempts to provide insights into client perspectives and perceptions of health care needs which should be requisite information for health care planners.

This book directly addresses a central issue concerning the benefits of articulating indigenous midwives with national health systems. The consideration of birth practices among the Bariba indicates that the degree to which patients and practitioners share models of clinical reality significantly affects patient perceptions of the quality of care received. Assumptions regarding sickness causation, concepts of diagnosis, and definitions of types of illness episodes are logically linked to treatment procedures and notions of what constitutes effective therapy. The reluctance of many rural Bariba women to select maternity clinics as a delivery option is largely due to the lack of homophily between parturients and clinic staff, and in particular, to different conceptions of the meaning of competent and effective obstetrical care.

If a primary public health goal in developing countries is to upgrade the quality of maternal and child health care, then it is useful to reconsider how a discrepancy between models of clinical reality held by patients and practitioners may constrain patients from utilizing available health care services. The degree to which patients and practitioners share assumptions regarding diagnosis and treatment, and expectations concerning appropriate role performance can be viewed in the context of the prevailing hierarchy of practitioners. Thus in the Bariba community, existing alternatives for obstetrical assistance might number the following:

Practitioners
doctor
nurse-midwive
nurse
trained indigenous midwife
indigenous midwife

"Hierarchy" refers here to stratification as it is perceived by government officials and by most peasant Bariba, who are sufficiently affected by the process of national integration to adopt such concepts of status differentiation, at least in terms of deference, if not preferred choice of treatment. The higher the position of the practitioner in the hierarchy, the greater the likely discrepancy between medical models held by rural patients and practitioners. This conclusion is amply illustrated in examples of obstetrical beliefs and practices which are widespread among Bariba women.

Handling of the placenta is a case in point. Both indigenous midwives, other indigenous healers and Bariba women share the belief that the placenta and the fetus "live" together in a sac suspended in the mother's abdomen. Because the two are thus attached within the mother's body, and because the placenta is believed to be part of the infant, the two should be delivered together. If the mother delivers the baby and the placenta does not follow within five or ten minutes, remedial action begins, in order to stimulate the expulsion of the placenta.

Midwives state that "it is the placenta which kills," and most indigenous birth attendants have a stock of treatments designed to treat a "delayed" placenta. These treatments range from sticking a feather down the throat of the parturient, gagging her with a porridge stick, feeding her medicines, rolling her abdomen with a broom or other object, and recourse to various ritual procedures. In fact, midwives have more treatments for expulsion of the placenta than for any other complications of delivery, indicating the perceived importance of this problem.

The interesting question here is what constitutes a retained placenta. Patients and indigenous practitioners share the fear that a placenta which is not delivered immediately is dangerous, and similarly, stories abound of women who have died or almost died because of complications associated with the placenta. Without attending a delivery, it is difficult to determine whether the placenta would be considered a "retained placenta" by cosmopolitan medical practitioners but it seems probable that many of the cases of allegedly retained placentas would not be considered medical problems in a maternity clinic or hospital.

The attitude of Beninois physicians who are aware of the procedures designed to treat a retained placenta is that some of the treatments such as rolling the parturient's abdomen with a broom may have the opposite effect to that which was intended. This indigenous practice, then, is not held to be therapeutic by nurses, nurse-midwives or physicians. Correspondingly, the assumptions which motivate treatments for the placenta are held to be false, although medical personnel do recognize the rationality of the concern for safe delivery of the placenta. It is rather the interpretation of "safe" and expectations regarding the ideal delivery, which differ. Rural clients share the assumptions of midwives and other indigenous healers regarding the potentially retained placenta but modes of diagnosis and treatment for this complication differ greatly between indigenous and cosmopolitan practitioners.

The effect of this discrepancy is that government medical personnel level criticisms and scorn at indigenous midwifery practices, and patients (and their relatives) worry that they are not receiving competent care when measures to extract the placenta are not commenced precipitously at deliveries attended by cosmopolitan practitioners. Where indigenous treatment fails to expel the placenta, women do seek clinic assistance. Nurse-midwives are known for their ability to do manual extractions which indigenous midwives usually do not attempt. The situation which may develop is that the patient has greater confidence in the indigenous procedures; therefore the matrone is the first resort.

If she fails, the parturient may arrive at a clinic or call for assistance but nurses and nurse-midwives possess stores of tales of women who hemorrhaged to death or died from other factors associated with delay in seeking "appropriate" treatment.

The folk illness *tigpiru* serves as a second example of differential interpretations of a pregnancy-related complaint. To Bariba, *tigpiru* is a condition prevalent among pregnant women. This sickness is conceptualized as redness which lies flat in the abdomen. As the sickness matures, it becomes round and protrudes through the anus or vagina. An additional symptom of *tigpiru* may be swollen limbs. Preferred treatment consists of fumigation with medicated substances or medicine to be ingested with sauce or porridge. Pregnant women with swollen legs, then, deduce that they are suffering from *tigpiru* and obtain appropriate medication from a matrone or other *tigpiru* specialist. Most women would not seek advice for swelling at a clinic. Those women who do attend prenatal consultations are often told to eliminate salt from their diet. However, even when the clinic midwife or her aide instruct women that eliminating salt will reduce oedema, patients tend to shrug at the lack of knowledgeability of the staff, who do not recognize that the real problem is *tigpiru*. Moreover, clinic staff tend to be unaware that some women who do try to reduce salt intake substitute potash or bicarbonate of soda as a sauce seasoning, thus counteracting the desired effect.

In considering women's utilization of maternity clinics, other culturally-specific interpretations of physiological concomitants of delivery are worth noting briefly. One is the notion of "long labor." Bariba women prefer to disguise signs of labor and criticize maternity clinics because staff observe patients in labor, thereby embarassing them. Women who do entertain the possibility of delivering at a clinic nonetheless prefer to arrive late in labor so they will not be obliged to wait under observation at the clinic. Pregnant women may also seek assistance in the event of long labor. The problematic issue is, as one matrone described it, that a courageous woman disguises her labor so that when others become aware, they think it is the initial stages of labor and much time remains, whereas in actuality, she is ready to deliver. A fearful woman, on the contrary, expresses pain and discomfort so soon after the onset of labor that those assisting her think her labor is long and problematic. Attempts to disguise signs of labor and even to obscure a long labor, in the case of a "courageous" woman, lead to the number of babies born en route to the clinic, or at home and brought to the clinic to be washed by the midwife.

In addition, the case of the prolapsed cord described in Chapter 7 demonstrated two significant points. First, that modesty constrains women from soliciting advice and assistance from one another – it defines boundaries for diagnosis and treatment in that the practitioner may not be allowed to examine the vaginal area. Second, where a witch birth or witch-proved abnormality is suspected, the clinic option is deferred to last resort. Furthermore, when

I urged the parturient to go to the clinic because I insisted on examining the "thing which came out," my diagnosis was later analyzed by the family to have derived from my touching the woman's abdomen, rather than from viewing the prolapsed cord. The significance in this episode is, it seems to me, that the observers perceived certain actions as efficacious, notably, my touching the woman, and ignored my suggestion that I could see that the cord was the problem. In this case the family chose to act on their interpretation of my diagnostic skills, and sent the woman to the district clinic with me. In another situation, the definition of the problem might have had the opposite effect.[34] To reiterate, interpretation of the event and corresponding recognition of dangers lead to decisions perceived as appropriate. However, both the problem under consideration and the ensuing decision may evoke discrepant evaluations from indigenous and cosmopolitan perspectives.

These examples taken from case studies of deliveries among Bariba women illustrate that (1) prospective maternity patients and Bariba indigenous practitioners share beliefs, values and role expectations to a greater extent than do Bariba patients and cosmopolitan medical personnel; and (2) this gulf between patients and practitioners deters woman from using clinics and leads to misunderstandings, anxieties and lack of compliance with instructions when women do choose the clinic option. In seeking to reduce this chasm and allow women to exploit the benefits of both indigenous and cosmopolitan medical systems, a policy approach favoring some form of accomodation or collaboration between the two systems is promising.

10.3. TRAINING PROGRAMS

To date, the government of Benin has experimented only tentatively with training programs for indigenous midwives. The Administration of the District of Kouande attempted two training sessions, one which sought to prepare literate teen-age girls to serve as obstetrical auxiliaries who would work primarily in dispensaries (1977) and a prior program which brought together the matrones of the district in an effort to teach them principles of hygiene and improved midwifery practices.

The program to train obstetrical auxiliaries has had meager results, primarily because village women did not approve of young, unmarried, childless obstetrical assistants, and the auxiliaries themselves were diffident and conscious of the culturally inappropriate role into which they had stepped. Similarly, the session to train the established matrones produced only antipathy and suspicion among the matrones, who claim they were insulted, mocked and inconvenienced by clinic staff. As a tangential effect of this experience, matrones who were asked to participate in the research on Bariba midwifery assumed that I, the researcher, was organizing a training program. They informed me adamantly that they would not leave their villages and go to another session.

Nonetheless, in spite of their negative experiences, and their grave suspicions concerning government officials, matrones did eventually express strong interest in supplementing their existing midwifery skills. Those matrones who participated in interviews and allowed me to observe deliveries with them increasingly requested information on complications of pregnancy and delivery with which they felt inadequate to cope. I found the matrones to be cognizant of their limitations and able to enumerate problems for which they lacked – but sought – solutions. This finding suggests that matrones would be receptive to learning new obstetrical techniques and practices; similarly, matrones might readily abandon practices which are potentially harmful, such as some measures to expel the placenta, upon learning substitute techniques. Certainly not all practicing matrones would be amenable to training. However, the attitude of Bariba matrones demonstrates that it is unwise to assume that matrones are too old, suspicious, secretive, or unintelligent to upgrade their midwifery techniques and practices.

This ethnographic study of maternity care in one African society provides support for the growing documentation of the benefits which may be gained from involving indigenous midwives in maternal and child health programs and underscores certain issues which require attention in any such efforts. Critical among these are ideological and structural barriers to the articulation of indigenous midwives (cf. Foster 1973: Chapters 4, 5, 6).

Ideological barriers: a primary barrier to involvement of midwives in the national health system in Benin, and one which threatens similar efforts in many developing nations, is the priority given to the premises of the cosmopolitan medical system. According to these premises, physicians and hospitals serve as the pivots of the system and the latest advances in medical technology are considered requisite. Public health goals may be subordinated to efforts in curative medicine. Correspondingly, reliance on indigenous healers and deterrence to indigenous medicine in general are incongruent with the medical model preferred at the national level. In contrast, at the local level, indigenous healers may react with indifference or suspicion to the concept of collaborating with a government program. This reaction may be based on negative experiences in prior interactions with government officials or on familiarity with government efforts to denigrate or abolish indigenous medicines as an option.

Structural barriers: a major problem which arises even where policy-makers advocate utilization of indigenous midwives is the lack of a systematic approach for articulating such healers with the national health system. Where, for example, will indigenous midwives be located in the hierarchy of medical practitioners? Are they to be considered collaborators or subordinates? What does "involvement" really mean? This may be an issue which needs to be examined on a case-by-case and country-by-country basis; however, in general it seems unreasonable to envisage indigenous healers and cosmopolitan practitioners sharing a body of knowledge to any large extent. An awareness of the difficulty of "integrating" healers in this sense has led to decisions, such as that taken in Benin, to bypass the indigenous midwives and train young, literate obstetrical auxiliaries who might more effectively be incorporated into the national health system. To what degree a sophisticated understanding of cosmopolitan medicine is necessary for an indigenous midwife to upgrade her skills remains unresolved.

An additional factor which may impede collaboration with midwives is the effect of class distinctions. Currently, national health personnel such as physicians and nurses tend to be drawn from the urban, western-educated elite, whereas healers are more often members of the peasantry. These class distinctions may serve to render both set of practitioners reluctant to collaborate. Moreover, in areas such as northern Benin, regionalism and ethnicity may also mitigate against collaboration between cosmopolitan practitioners and indigenous healers. Ideological and structural barriers notwithstanding, the Bariba experience indicates that it is worthwhile to attempt to address these problematic issues. In general, the Bariba data suggests several policy recommendations.

(1) Given the limited number of western-trained obstetrical personnel in developing nations, especially in rural Africa, it seems reasonable to maximize available medical resources by using the skills of indigenous midwives. In Benin the ratio of government midwives to population was one per 12,890 as recently as 1977; and there was only one nurse per 3,220 inhabitants. In comparison, in the District of Kouande, I estimate that there is at least one matrone per 200 inhabitants (calculations include only the best-known practitioners.) Clearly, then, a system which incorporates the skills of both matrones and cosmopolitan medical professionals would greatly improve the ratio of health care providers to population in need.

The most pertinent role for the trained midwife would be to provide a first level of screening and referral; thus the goal of training would be to teach the birth attendant to detect pathology by the most simple parameters possible, recognizing that some seemingly minor changes could have major effects on morbidity and mortality. This role would build on the interest of the midwife in offering competent service to her clients but would not necessarily require her to work in close collaboration with cosmopolitan medical practitioners or to undergo sophisticated training. In fact the scope of training for midwives should be limited to a necessary minimum, and changes should be evaluated in terms of "appropriate technology;" in other words, techniques and practices should be based on a pragmatic appraisal of existing resources. It is evident, for example, that in Benin, where only capital city clinics currently are well-stocked with drugs, equipment and personnel, that it would not be productive to train midwives to rely on unavailable supplies or support. An efficiently functioning referral system cannot, for instance, rely at present on motorized vehicles in a setting where gasoline supplies are undependable and the cost of purchasing and maintaining sufficient vehicles would be prohibitive. In sum, devising a workable training course which both improves the obstetrical competence of the midwives and conforms to the cultural context is a task which might best be shared by anthropologists, policy planners, biomedical specialists, and indigenous practioners.

(2) In the long-run, certain aspects of traditional care such as delivery position, traditional pharmacopeia, and modes of psychological support might be advantageous to maintain. Moreover, the advantages of hospital delivery over home delivery need to be seriously reconsidered, given local conditions and prevailing attitudes, both of which may change over time.[34] Thus as long as clinics and hospitals are ill-stocked, sporadically staffed, and inaccessible to much of the intended target population, efforts to improve maternal and child health care might well focus on safer home deliveries and on an effective screening and referral system.

(3) The attitudes of civil servants in the health service and indigenous midwives toward one another are often characterized by lack of mutual respect, and sometimes by condescension on the part of the civil servants and by fear on the part of the midwives. It seems to me that midwives will respond to the acknowledgement by the civil servants of a situation of mutual need, since health professionals need the midwife, who is integrated into the local community and has invaluable ties and knowledge. The midwife is the base of the referral system and although she may perceive her role as subordinate, because she is referring "up" in the status hierarchy, she is a necessary collaborator. Regardless of her lack of a certain body of knowledge, one can respect the indigenous midwife for her years of experience and for her competence in the traditional pharmacopeia.

(4) Training is most likely to be well-received and pursued if it is based on an in-depth study of customary beliefs and practices and if it addresses issues known to be of interest to midwives and their clients, as well as the routine concerns of the modern health system. In addition, cosmopolitan health services such as maternity clinics would provide improved care and consistently attract a large client population if cultural factors were recognized as significant to health care delivery. Clinic personnel might, for instance, routinely inquire of patients their perceptions of the problem under consideration in order to better offer acceptable suggestions for diagnosis and treatment. By this approach, national health service practitioners can begin to address the problems inherent in the differing views of medical reality held by themselves and their clients.

(5) Finally, midwives need to be seen as the true "brokers" they are:

(a) as obstetrical specialists, they serve an intermediate or mediating function in bringing babies into the world;

(b) as midwives trained in government programs, they can serve a mediating role between Bariba culture and the non-Bariba world – literally, they operate to integrate Bariba into the world beyond the District of Kouande.

I am arguing, then, that structural and ideological barriers to the involvement of indigenous midwives in national health systems can be surmounted. The Bariba research validates the contention that a national health delivery system must respond to client perspectives on health and illness in order to achieve optimal effect and to function as a preferred choice of health care. I have suggested that obstetrical decisions are not capricious or precipitous, but rather, are the outcome of cultural expectations, within which context options are assessed and selected. An effective health care system must take into account the assumptions of the client population which form the basis of health care goals. Moreover, such a system must mesh the perceived health care needs of the indigenous population with the premises and objectives of cosmopolitan medicine. The magnitude of this task is impressive but the direction nonetheless imperative.

APPENDICES

APPENDIX A: DEMOGRAPHIC DATA

TABLE 26
Age structure of Pehunko according to census*

	Ages						
Neighborhood	16–20	21–25	26–30	31–35	36–40	41+	Total
Sinawararou	18	12	15	12	19	12	88
Pehunko Center	10	16	33	14	10	8	91
Gbankerou	0	1	2	0	3	1	7
Tance	1	2	5	1	4	3	16
Total #	29	31	55	27	36	24	202
%	14	15	27	13	18	12	

compared to

Age structure of survey of women of reproductive age**

	Ages						
	16–20	21–25	26–30	31–35	36–40	41+	Total
Total #	15	26	26	19	19	15	120
%	13	22	22	16	16	13	

* I am grateful to Harry Raulet for assisting me with the analysis of this demographic data.
** The age structure of the sample of women of reproductive age is comparable to that of women in Pehunko as officially listed in the census except in the categories of women aged 21–25 and 26–30. However, taken those two categories in aggregate, assuming ages 21–30 as a prime childbearing period, the discrepancy diminished (village = 42%; sample = 44%).

TABLE 27
Official census and research sample

	# Households	Mean size	S.D.
Official census	60	14.96	15.70
Research sample	79	14.36	8.45

TABLE 28
Proportion of live births ending in infant or child death

Age at interview*	# Intervews	Livebirths ending in death		
		# deceased	# live births	%
15–20	15	2	17	12
21–25	26	9	47	19
26–30	26	17	89	19
31–35	19	22	87	25
36–40	19	35	122	29
41+	15	37	108	34
Totals	120	122	470	26

Other pertinent data:

Total number of pregnancies of sample	520
Pregnancy wastage, including stillbirths	50
Mean number of pregnancies	8
Mean number of live births	7

* Age structure of sample closely reflects actual age structure of village; see Table 25. (note 30)

APPENDIX B: FEMALE CIRCUMCISION SONGS

I.

Biibe yoriyo surukpɛ wori basiyo surukpe
(no glutinous sauce together with "that which hurts")

Munɔnu basiyo surukpe ka samtunsunɔ̃ surukpɛ
(no tree with red flowers/with that which hurts/ . . . with non-glutinous sauce . . . is good)

II.

Bɛsɛsa kara bee goo somburu siare
(we never congratulate anyone for working: interpreted as –
circumcisers don't congratulate others because they do so well themselves)

Bo gogube goo n bu bwĩyare
(no one hits a wound: interpreted as –
don't seek quarrels)

Baru woo gogube goo baro karare
(a pushing person pushes someone)

Bɛsɛsa Doh wɔworu sãra yĩo
(we have confidence in the Land Chief of Doh; from the Circumcision Song of the Village of Doh)

III. (also sung at marriages and at the death of a hunter)

mɔkpɛbwɛ̃bwɛ̃ra mɔkpɛ
(fermented corn paste is poverty)

An gu tausunobɛnum ma
(if you die in war it is because of fear)

An gu yebu sonu yikura
(if you die while making yam mounds it is laziness)

Bɛnum ma saka nɔ̃ɔ sɔɔ wa wɔllɔ
(fear makes a bad mood)

Yikura sa ka nɔ̃ɔ sɔɔ wa gbã me
(it is laziness which makes us grimace)

NOTES

1. Accurate demographic data are unavailable for the District of Kouande. However, the district population is estimated at approximately 18,000. Given a crude birth rate of about 50, one would expect 800–900 births per year in the district. This would suggest that from 25 to 30% of district deliveries occurred in the maternity clinic. However, it seems probable that the district population is greatly underestimated. Moreover, use of the clinic is heavily limited to the district seat. It would be unwarranted, then, to conclude that 25% of the women in the district utilize the maternity clinic for deliveries. A more conclusive estimation of clinic utilization will be possible subsequent to the United Nations census currently in progress.
2. "Bariba" is a Europeanized term possibly derived from the Yoruba name "Bariba" used to refer to the population who call themselves *Baatɔnu* (plural *Baatɔmbu*) (Lombard 1965:43). Writers such as Lombard (1965) and Baldus (1974) have referred to the *Baatɔmbu* as *Baatɔmba*, however here I am adopting the plural *Baatɔmbu* as cited by the National Dahomean Commission for Linguistics, Publications No. 2 and No. 4.

   In this discussion I am using the term Bariba when referring to the *Baatɔmbu* because it is the term currently utilized by the government of the People's Republic of Benin and in Nigeria and by which the Baatɔmbu are best known in the literature.
3. The terms homophily and heterophily are awkward, thus causing me some discomfiture. Nonetheless, this terminology is current in research addressing similar topics to my own and having no desire to invent new jargon, I have decided to retain the terms used by Rogers and Shomemaker.
4. "Civil servant" in the context of this discussion refers to public sector employees (those paid by the national government); this category includes all government administrators and personnel, such as Ministry officials working both at the national and local levels; bank employees; post employees; and all health personnel including nurses and nurse-midwives who are trained in national schools in the capital and posted throughout the country by the Ministry of Health. The Civil Service also includes the Agriculture Service, including local officials such as village-level extension agents and sub-district extension officers.

   Benin (Dahomey until 1974) has long been noted for the disproportionate percentage of its budget allocated to the public sector. Thus in 1970, 80% of the national revenues went towards salaries of civil servants and 'agents of the state,' who numbered approximately 29,000 in a population estimated at 2.9 million. (Survey of African Economics, Vol. 3, International Monetary Fund. Washington: 1970).

   In order to understand the position of civil servants in a northern district such as Kouande (and in the province of the Atakora as a whole), it is necessary to recognize that during the colonial period, the French presence was oriented towards the south of the country (Ronen 1975:37, 64). Compared with other French colonies, there was a great interest in education in Dahomey and the country later acquired fame because of its intellectuals, who served in the colonial administration throughout French West Africa (Ronen 1975:65). However, there has always been a significantly unequal distribution in school attendance between the north and south, a reflection of a general social, cultural and political dichotomy between northern and southern regions. Thus in 1948 about 32,000 children attended school in Dahomey of whom about 2,900 were from northern ethnic groups. Even in the north, 90% of the students were from the south. This in turn has resulted in a situation where the majority of civil servants have been southerners and correspondingly, it is southerners who represent the salaried elite of the country (although this situation is changing as more efforts are made by the national government to provide educational opportunities to northerners and to enforce compulsory education requirements).

Civil servants, then, have traditionally been considered foreigners by northerners. As Ronen states in discussing southern teachers, a southern official was rejected by a northern population because " . . . he belonged, together with Europeans, to a different *race* . . . . A similar attitude existed on the part of the southerners toward their northern compatriots . . . ." (67). This situation has affected utilization of health facilities and maternity clinics in particular in that health personnel, as southerners, have traditionally been perceived both as "foreigners" and as members of the elite and were rarely integrated into local society. This situation has been modified somewhat in recent years in the Kouande area as southern officials married Bariba women, and as the national government presence has become more evident in all aspects of Bariba life (e.g., agricultural operations, marketing, "ideological orientation sessions," compulsory education, literacy campaigns, immunization campaigns, and so forth).

5. The Bariba conception of the supreme deity seems similar to that described by Herskovits for the Fon of southern Benin. Like Gusunɔ̃, the Fon deity Mawu is believed to have created the world and her will determines its ultimate destiny. She orders the life and death of every individual although she herself must abide by "rules that control supernatural as well as human behavior" (Herskovits 1967:292). Herskovits comments on the supposition that in African religion the Creator leaves the world to "its own devices and to the pleasures of inferior Gods" (289). Looking beyond superficial indicators, he suggests that Mawu is, in fact, not far removed from participation in the universe. Similarly, the Bariba deity *Gusunɔ̃* can be approached and induced to act on an individual's behalf. However, it is my impression that various spirits are of more immediate concern to Bariba than is *gusunɔ̃*.
6. In any event the importance of divination among the Bariba is in no way comparable to the significance of Fa divination among the Fon, of whom Herskovits states that "throughout the discussion of Dahomean life there has been no phase where the necessity of consulting the diviner before taking any action is taken has not been stressed" (Herskovits 1967:305). Similarly, among the Yoruba, Ifa divination (from which the Fon divination derives) provides knowledge of what destiny lies in store for a person. Ifa determines which deity a person should worship, which sacrifices may be necessary, the appropriate occupation for a person to follow. Ifa divination gives warnings against mystical dangers and in case of any misfortune, Ifa is consulted (Bascom 1969:118). The Bariba do rely on divination for interpretation of problematic events and for guidance; however, the Bariba do not have a system of divination as complex or of as pervasive application as Fa or Ifa.
7. A qualification to this statement is necessary: I found that many people recognized the Bariba name of the plants and other botanicals recommended for treatment of obstetrical complications. Often people were not aware that the item in question could be used for obstetrical care, but did know of other uses for it. This was generally the case of botanicals other than for obstetrical care – the same item was utilized for different purposes by differing people, although some plants or barks were widely known for one particular cure. Therefore, although I can say that some medicinal preparations seemed to be used only for the purpose recommended by a midwife, probably other individuals would recognize at least a component of the preparation as useful for other disorders. I should add that most midwives were adamant that the medicine prescribed would only be effective for the function indicated. For example, I assumed that a medicine which would accelerate labor would act (or be presumed to act) by increasing or strengthening contractions. I expected that the same medicine, by producing the same effect would also expel the placenta or possibly, provoke an abortion. The midwives

denied that one medicine would be effective to accomplish different *purposes* (i.e., placenta, delivery of fetus, expulsion of fetus) and that each medicine had its own identity and function.

8. The importance of fecundity and motherhood in rural Africa has been widely documented (cf. Paulme 1960:14; Gessain 1969:34.)
9. "His spiritual power which authorized him to manipulate the most dangerous natural element, fire, and to fabricate all the instrument which had power of life – agricultural tools – as well as of death – arms." (My translation)
10. "Each attitude of daily life tended always to specify a status and there was no contact between individuals which was not, first of all, for one, recognition of his hierarchical inferiority, if not his dependency." (My translation)
11. In a discussion of formal political positions such as this, it is useful to note Lebeuf's comment that "In all the political systems which have either one or two women at the top of the hierarchy, these women belong to a very respected group drawn from a social class which already confers on them, even before they occupy their special roles, rights and privileges which are in marked contrast to those of the rest of the female population" (Lebeuf 1960:9).
12. "Potters, midwives, initiates (of spirit cults) and above all, cult priestesses had an influence which often surpassed the limits of the village or even the region, and certain reputations might spread throughout the Bariba country, by the intermediary of the praise-singers." (My translation)
13. In this discussion, power and authority are defined following M. G. Smith: "Authority is, in the abstract, the right to make a particular decision and to command obedience . . . Power . . . is the ability to act effectively on persons or things, to make or secure favourable decisions which are not of right allocated to the individuals or their roles" (quoted in Rosaldo and Lamphere 1974:21).
14. The reasons why no market women's associations exist in the rural Bariba region are not germane to this discussion. However, it is interesting to note that in Leis' discussion of Ijaw women's associations, she suggests that women's associations are most likely to be found where certain conditions are present. These include: patrilocality, patriliny, polygyny, permanent villages, a market system, and economic independence among women derived from the trade and market complex. Other factors such as diffuse loyalties of both sexes, or situations where women are strongly oriented towards their own kin, may inhibit the development of non-kin-based women's associations (Leis 1974). All the conditions favorable to association formation are present in Bariba society. Possibly among rural Bariba women, the lack of organization results from women's orientation towards their own paternal and maternal kin ("a woman is always a stranger in her husband's house"); a sparse population in the region in spite of permanent villages; difficulties in transportation and communication. The fact that most women, operating as individuals, engage in petty trade and do not amass a large capital may also be a factor.
15. It is evident that all professional specialization, especially that concerning fecundity and birth, supplemented the prestige and strengthened the special status of women.
16. Correspondingly, the curse of sterility is evident in the burial procedures for a person who dies without offspring. Such a person is beaten in the area of the lower back and buried facing west, the direction of sorrow and obscurity, in the hope that such a grave misfortune will never afflict others in the society. In a sense, burial of a barren person is comparable to excommunication – the cursed individual is banished from the community of the healthy and the blessed and deemed no longer to exist.
17. Men are rarely present at births but in dangerous deliveries, if witchcraft is suspected, a powerful male healer (generalist) may be called.
18. For this computation, it was assumed that when asked for "number of pregnancies," matrones reported live births. Matrones contrasted with non-matrones as follows:

Women over age 40

$$\frac{\text{Deceased children}}{\text{Live births}} = 34\%$$

Matrones (all 40+)

$$\frac{\text{Deceased children}}{\text{Live births}} = 24\%$$

19. In Bariba society, the father's sister/brother's daughter relationship is traditionally one of respect and awe in that the father's sister's curse can result in sterility. However, the father's curse is balanced by her power to bless and to allow fertility of her brother's daughter whereas there is a taboo against the parturient's mother being present at the delivery particularly for the delivery of the daughter's first child. This taboo might be explained in terms of the "social equivalence" of mothers and daughters and the idea that same sex offspring are inherently replacements for their parents. Thus the childbearing activity of a mother's own offspring is the death knell for the mother and her generation and the parturient's own mother must avoid viewing her own replacement in the act of giving birth. The vagina may be perceived as the symbol of the production of children and the quintessence of the social identity of a woman and correspondingly, the parturient's mother must not look upon her daughter's vagina in the very act of reproducing. (Based on personal communication with Dr. Robert McKinley.)
20. See Keesing 1973 for a discussion of composite of social identity.
21. Cults were in very low profile during the research period due to government restrictions on their functioning (see Chapter 11) which restricted data collection on such topics as internal organization of cults and cult politics.
22. Given the attitude of Bariba women towards childbirth and the stoicism observed at deliveries, I would suspect that the fact that 60% of the sample did have someone present indicates a high rate of complications, rather than a lack of effort in adhering to the ideal.
23. It is impossible to obtain data on numbers of witch babies actually killed due to the fact that this topic of questioning does not lend itself to survey research. However, elderly and young informants alike claim that witch babies are not allowed to live. Some witch babies, especially babies born with teeth, are an exception in that they may be given to the Fulbe to raise; these children formerly constituted a category of slave called *mareyobu* by Bariba.

    The *mareyobou* (or *machube*, in Fulfulde) were studied by Baldus who notes that the belief that the child whose first teeth appear in the upper gums brings disaster, illness and death to its family is a belief found in other areas of West Africa, for example, among the Yoruba of eastern Dahomey and Nigeria. Meek reports similar practices among the Ibo (Meek 1937:290–291). "It seems, however, that nowhere else was the belief taken as seriously as among the Batomba [Bariba] and nowhere else did it lead to the same elaborate protective measures" (Baldus 1974:361).

    According to Baldus, the alternative measures taken were to have the child killed by the *gossiko* (burial official); to have the child raised as a slave by the *gossiko*; or after the pastoral Fulbe moved into the area in the 18th and early 19th centuries, such children were given to them to be raised and kept as slaves. These children were fully integrated into Fulbe family life but never lost the identity of a dangerous child abandoned by the Batomba. Of these *machube*, Baldus writes "Of all slave groups in Borgou with the possible exception of the *gandogibu* [who were the property of Bariba aristocrats] the *machube* were the most openly exploited as an economic asset" (Baldus 1974:362). Similarly, Lombard remarks that these slaves were ranked at the bottom of the slave hierarchy.

24. Snow 1974 further documents this point.
25. According to the World Health Organization, "the percentage of estimated deliveries attended by Traditional Birth Attendants in several developing countries varied from 60 to over 80% in 1972" (WHO Publication 18, 1975:14). The Bariba, then, correspond to sectors of rural populations in other developing countries in not relying on cosmopolitan medical services for maternity care. They differ in the extent to which women idealize the "solitary delivery."
26. The hospital file of one woman who informed me that she had *tigpiru* listed her condition as "giant prolapsed genitals" [French translation].

    The *New American Pocket Dictionary* defines these terms as follows:

prolapse:	the falling of a structure
prolapsed uterus:	uterus descends into the vagina and may be visible at the vaginal orifice.
cystocele:	prolapse of the posterior wall of the urinary bladder into the anterior vaginal wall
rectocele:	prolapse of the rectum so that it lies outside the anus

27. Fabrega and Tyma offer another perspective on the cross-cultural study of pain. They seek a way of conceptualizing how language and culture influence the experiences a person has during disease and choose pain as one attribute of the disease experience " . . . which implicates mind-body relations . . . ." (Fabrega and Tyma 1976a:349). They argue that "cross-cultural linguistic studies are needed which will carefully document perceptual, behavioral and cognitive features of 'pain' and of other signals of disease" (p. 349).

    The authors suggest that pain behaviors "embrace changes in facial expression, demeanor and activity. They also include verbalizations which describe and qualify the pain experience in a determinate way. The latter constitutes the *linguisitic* dimension of pain, i.e., the structure and content of verbal descriptions of pain" (Fabrega and Tyma 1976a: 350). They then ask how pain is given meaning and significance by means of language. Unfortunately, I cannot add to the discussion on this topic, having insufficient data on terms used in Bariba to describe pain. I plan to obtain more information on Bariba pain vocabulary in a future research project.
28. One brief article of interest related to this topic is Davitz et al. 1976, on "Suffering As Viewed in Six Different Cultures." This article reports on a study regarding nurses in six cultures; nurses were asked to judge the amount of physical pain and psychological distress patients were experiencing. The study indicates that nurses, reflecting the cultural system in which they live, vary markedly in their perceptions regarding patient suffering. For example, Americans believed Oriental patients felt less pain than patients from other ethnic backgrounds whereas Oriental nurses believe their Oriental patients are especially sensitive to physical pain (p. 1297). The authors note that "These results probably reflect cultural differences in the relationship between experience and expressive behavior . . . in the Japanese culture, strong feelings are not necessarily expressed by overt behavior" (p. 1237).
29. Fabrega and Tyma distinguish between pain which has no readily visible source or basis and pain resulting from traumatic or visible changes or events which impinge on the body (e.g., childbirth). They suggest that "many such 'visible' bodily changes when expected or planned for may not be dealt with conceptually as pain at all." (Fabrega and Tyma 1976a:350) It is my impression that Bariba do conceptualize the sensations of childbirth as pain – the appropriate *response*, however, is "absence of manifest behavior."
30. An accurate assessment of distance as a factor influencing clinic utilization requires census data which are not obtainable for all of the villages cited in the discussions.

These data are necessary in order to determine the ratio of clinic users from each village of origin to population size of the respective villages. If distance is an influential factor, the above percentages decrease with distance from the clinic site. A sample of villages for which population has been estimated is presented in Table 25.

TABLE 25
Ratio of clinic users to village size in relation to distance traveled

Village	Distance	Clinic users 1976–77	Estimated village population	%*
Kouande	0	199	3,100	6.4
Gbeke	6	4	838	0.4
Orou-Kayo	9	8	1,355	0.5
Sekeguru	9	2	834	0.2
Ganikperu	12	0	1,325	0.0
Kagare	14	0	361	0.0
Makru	16	0	502	0.0
Tiku	16	0	1,044	0.0
Niassera	17	1	706	0.1
Niarusu	17	0	631	0.0
Niaro	18	0	532	0.0
Maka	18	0	421	0.0
Kouba	21	0	759	0.0
Pehunko	37	3	2,114	0.1
Yemasson	59	1	834	0.1

* $\frac{\text{Number Users}}{\text{Village Size}} = \%$.

The above table indicates that percentages do roughly decrease with distance. However, I do not have the necessary data to differentiate distance as a factor from the effect of other factors such as type of village (e.g., percent of civil servants or traders in the population); a distinction might, for example, be pertinent in the case of Pehunko. In general, however, the above findings are not inconsistent with the hypothesis that distance is at least a contributing factor to the use pattern described.

31. "Emic" refers to analysis based on categories elicited from members of a culture themselves whereas "etic" is a term used for analyses based on categories derived from the western scientific traditions. Sometimes these concepts are colloquially referred to as "inside" and "outside" views.
32. See, for example, Ademuwagun et al. 1979, "Part III: The Interaction Between African and Western Medicine," for discussion of the benefits and means of collaboration between indigenous and cosmopolitan systems. Tolani Asuni presents a more skeptical perspective on the merits of indigenous healers in Rubel and Sargent (eds.) 1979.
33. The World Health Organization has engaged in considerable deliberations regarding the role of midwifery personnel in developing countries (cf. WHO Publication #18, 1975; #44, 1979). In discussing the benefits of involving traditional birth attendants in national health systems, a WHO publication on the traditional birth attendant suggests "articulating," rather than "integrating" the services of the TBA with the national health system. The establishment of informal links between the "organized health system" and the TBA is intended to avoid loss of identity for the birth attendants (1979:8). The document urges that

. . . the concern should not centre on integrating the TBA into the modern system but rather on ensuring that, within the TBA as a person, modern and traditional concepts and modes of practice are so integrated as to eliminate only traditional practices and rituals that are clearly shown to be harmful, and to instill only modern concepts and techniques that are absolutely essential to the safety of the persons under the care of the TBA" (8).

34. See Snow 1974:94 for a discussion of an episode with similar implications among Black Americans.
35. In addition to the Benin information, other studies suggest that there is little evidence that hospital delivery is always safer than delivery at home (Population Reports May 1980:J-449).

BIBLIOGRAPHY

Ademuwagun, Z. A., Ayoade, John A. A., Harrison, Ira E., and Dennis M. Warren (eds.)
1979 African Therapeutic Systems. Waltham, Mass.: Crossroads Press.

Alland, A., Jr.
1970 Adaptation in Cultural Evolution: An Approach to Medical Anthropology. New York and London: Columbia University Press.

Asuni, T.
1979 The Dilemma of Traditional Healing with Special Reference to Nigeria. Social Science and Medicine (Special Issue): Parallel Medical Systems: Papers from a Workshop on "The Healing Process." 13B(1):33–41.

Baldus, B.
1974 Social Structure and Ideology: Cognitive and Behavioral Responses to Servitude Among the Machube of Northern Dahomey. Canadian Journal of African Studies 8(2):355–83.

Barth, F.
1967 On the Study of Social Change. American Anthropologist 69(6):661–69.

Barth, F.
1969 Models of Social Organization. Occasional Paper No. 23, Royal Anthropologist Institute of Great Britain and Ireland.

Bascom, William
1969 Ifa Divination: Communication Between Gods and Men in West Africa. Bloomington: Indiana Univ. Press.

Billington, W. R. et al.
1963 Custom and Child Health in Buganda III. Pregnancy and Childbirth. Tropical and Geographical Medicine 15:134–37.

Blau, P. M.
1964 Exchange and Power in Social Life. New York: Wiley.

Buchler, I. R. and H. A. Selby
1968 Kinship and Social Organization: An Introduction to Theory and Method. New York: Macmillan.

Cancian, F.
1966 Maximization as Norm, Strategy and Theory: A Comment on Programmatic Statements in Economic Anthropology American Anthropologist 68:465–70.

Chelly, M.
1976 Integration of the Traditional Midwives into the Tunisian Family Planning Programme. Paper presented to the National Conference on Nigerian Women and Development in Relation to Changing Family Structure. University of Ibadan, Nigeria, April 26–30.

Cohen, M. D., J. C. March, and J. P. Olsen
1972 A Garbage Can Model of Organizational Choice. Administrative Science Quarterly 17(1):1–26.

Collier, J. F.
1974 Women in Politics. *In* Woman, Culture and Society, M. Z. Rosaldo and L. Lamphere (eds.), Stanford: Stanford University Press.

Colson, A. C.
1971 The Differential Use of Medical Resources in Developing Countries. Journal of Health and Social Behavior 12:226–37.

Commission Nationale Dahomeenne de Linguistique #2
1974 Guide de Lecture Bariba. Berne, Commission Nationale Suisse pour l'UNESCO.
Commission Nationale Dahomeenne de Linguistique #4
1974 Abrégé de Grammaire Bariba. Parakou, Editions "Presses du Borgou."
Cosminsky, S.
1976 Cross-Cultural Perspectives on Midwifery. *In* Medical Anthropology, F. X. Grollig, S. J. Haley, and H. B. Haley (ed.), Paris and The Hague: Mouton Publishers.
Davenport-Slack, S. and C. H. Boylan
1974 Psychological Correlates of Childbirth Pain. Psychosomatic Medicine 36(3):215–23.
Davitz, L. et al.
1976 Suffering as Viewed in Six Different Cultures. American Journal of Nursing 76(8): 1296–97.
Donabedian, A.
1972 Models for Organizing the Delivery of Personal Health Services and Criteria for Evaluating Them. Milbank Memorial Fund Quarterly 50 (part 2), (October): 103–53.
Ekanem, R. et al.
1975 The Role of Traditional Birth Attendants in the South Eastern State of Nigeria. IPMS Publication No. 3. University of Ife, Faculty of Social Sciences.
Flwood, P. C.
1973 Evaluation of the Clinical Importance of Anemia. The American Journal of Clinical Nutrition 26:958–64.
Erasmus, C. L.
1952 Changing Folk Beliefs and the Relativity of Empirical Knowledge. Southwestern Journal of Anthropology 8:411–28.
Evans-Pritchard, E. E.
1937 Witchcraft, Oracles and Magic Among and Azande. Oxford: Clarendon Press.
Fabrega, Horacio Jr.
1974 Disease and Social Behavior an Interdisciplinary Perspective. Cambridge, Mass.: The MIT Press.
Fabrega, Horacio Jr. and Stephen Tyma
1976a Language and Cultural Influences in the Description of Pain. British J. Med. Psychol. 49:49–371.
Fabrega, Horacio Jr. and Stephen Tyma
1976b Culture, Language and the Shaping of an Illness: An Illustration Based on Pain. J. of Psychosomatic Research 20:323–337.
Ferguson, J. C. et al.
1968 Anemia in Nairobi Region. East African Medical Journal 45(10):663–76.
Fikry, M.
1977 Preliminary Report: Traditional Maternal and Child Health Care and Related Problems in the Sahel. A bibiliographic study. USAID.
Firth, R.
1967 Themes in Economic Anthropology: A General Comment. *In* Themes in Economic Anthropology, R. Firth (ed.), London, Tavistock.
Ford, C. S.
1945 A Comparative Study of Human Reproduction. 1964 edition. Yale University Publications in Anthropology #32. Human Relations Area File Press.
Foster, G. M.
1958 Problems in Intercultural Health Practice. Pamphlet 12. New York, Social Science Research Council.
Foster, G. M.
1962 Traditional Societies and Technological Change. 1973 edition. New York, Harper and Row, Publishers.

Foster, G. M. and B. G. Anderson
1978 Medical Anthropology. New York, San Francisco, Academic Press.
Frankel, Barabra
1977 Childbirth in the Ghetto: Folk Beliefs of Negro Women in a North Philadelphia Hospital Ward. San Francisco: R. E. Research Associates, Inc.
Frankenberg and Leeson
1976 Disease, Illness and Sickness: Social Aspects of the Choice of Healer in a Lusaka Suburb. *In* Social Anthropology and Medicine, J. B. Loudon (ed.), London, New York, San Francisco: Academic Press.
Frazer, J.
1922 The Golden Bough. Abridged edition. London: Macmillan and Co.
Freedman, D. et al.
1978 Statistics. New York: W. V. Norton and Company, Inc.
Freedman, L. and V. Ferguson
1950 The Question of "Painless Childbirth" in Primitive Cultures. American Journal of Orthopsychiatry 20(2):363–72.
Gardezi, H. N. and A. Inayatullah
1969 The Dai Study. Lahore, West Pakistan Family Planning Association.
Garn, S. M., N. J. Smith, and D. C. Clark
1975 The Magnitude and the Implications of Apparent Race Differences in Hemoglobin Values. The American Journal of Clinical Nutrition 28:563–68.
Geertz, C.
1966 Religion as a Cultural System. *In* Anthropological Approaches to the Study of Religion, M. Banton (ed.), London: Tavistock Publications Ltd.
Gessain, M.
1960 Coniagui Women. *In* Women in Tropical Africa, D. Paulme (ed.), Berkeley: University of California Press.
Gillies, E.
1976 Causal Criteria in African Classifications of Disease. *In* Social Anthropology and Medicine, J. B. Loudon (ed.), London, New York, San Francisco: Academic Press.
Glick, L.
1967 Medicine as a Ethnographic Category: The Gimi of the New Guinea Highlands. Ethnology 6(1):31–56.
Gluckman, M. and E. Devons
1964 Conclusions: Modes and Consequences of Limiting a Field of Study. *In* Closed Systems and Open Minds: The Limits of Naivety in Social Anthropology, M. Gluckman (ed.), Edinburgh and London: Oliver and Boyd.
Good, Charles, John M. Hunter, Selig H. Katz, and Sidney S. Katz
1979 The Interface of Dual Systems of Health Care in the Developing World Toward Health Policy Initiatives in Africa. Soc. Sci and Med. 13D:141–154.
Goodenough, W.
1956 Residence Rules. Southwestern Journal of Anthropology 12:22–37.
Gould, H. A.
1957 The Implications of Technological Change for Folk and Scientific Medicine. American Anthropologist 59:507–16.
Grollig, F. X., S. J. and Harold B. Haley (eds.)
1976 Medical Anthropology. The Hague and Paris: Mouton.
Hanks, J. R.
1963 Maternity and Its Rituals in Bang Chan. Cornell Thailand Project Interim Report Series #6. Ithaca, New York, Cornell University Press.
Hardy, J. D. and C. T. Javert
1949 Studies on Pain: Measurements of Pain Intensity in Childbirth. Journal of Clinical Investigation 28:153–62.

Harrison, Ira E.
1979 Traditional Healers: A Neglected Source of Health Manpower. *In* Ademuwagun et al. (eds.), African Therapeutic Systems, Waltham: Crossroads Press.
Heath, A.
1976 Rational Choice and Social Exchange. Cambridge, Cambridge University Press.
Herskovits, Melville J.
1967 Dahomey. An Ancient West African Kingdom Vol. II. Evanston: Northwestern University Press.
Hilgard, E. R. and J. R. Hilgard
1975 Hypnosis in the Relief of Pain. Los Altos: William Kaufmann.
Homans, G. C.
1961 Social Behavior: Its Elementary Forms. London: Routledge and Kegan Paul.
Howard, A.
1963 Land, Activiity Systems and Decision-Making Models in Rotuma. Ethnology 2:407–40.
Jafarety, L. A. et al.
1968 Use of Medical, Para-Medical and Traditional Midwives in the Pakistan Family Planning Program. Demography 5(2):666–78.
Janzen, J. M.
1978 The Quest for Therapy in Lower Zaire. Berkeley: University of California Press.
Javert, C. T. and J. T. Hardy
1950 Measurement of Pain Intensity in Labor and Its Physiologic, Neurologic, and Pharmacologic Implications. American Journal of Obstetrics and Gynecology 60:552–63.
Jett, J.
1977 The Role of Traditional Midwives in the Modern Health Sector in West and Central Africa USAID Report.
Jordan, B.
1978 Birth in Four Cultures. Montreal and St. Albans, Vermont: Eden Press.
Keesing, R. M.
1967 Statistical Models and Decision-Models of Social Structure: A Kwaio Case. Ethnology: 1–16.
Keesing, R. M.
1973 Toward a Model of Role Analysis. *In* A Handbook of Method in Cultural Anthropology, R. Naroll and R. Cohen (eds.), New York: Columbia University Press.
Kelly, J.
1967 The Influences of Native Customs on Obstetrics in Nigeria. Obstetrics and Gynecology 30(4):608–12.
Kiteme, Kamuti
1976 Traditional African Medicine. *In* F. X. Grollig, S. J., Harold B. Haley (eds.), Medical Anthropology. The Hague: Mouton.
Kleinman, Arthur, Leon Eisenberg, and Byron Good
1978a Culture, Illness, and Care. Clinical Lessons from Anthropologic and Cross-Cultural Research. Annals of Internal Medicine 88(2):251–258.
Kleinman, Arthur
1978b Comparisons of Practitioner-patient Interactions in Taiwan: The Cultural Construction of Clinical Reality. *In* Culture and Healing in Asian Societies, Kleinman et al. (eds.), Boston: Hall.
Kluckhohn, F. and F. L. Strodtbeck
1961 Variations in Value Orientations. Evanston: Row, Peterson and Co.
Knottenbelt, J. D.
1973 An Investigation into the Incidence and Nature of Anaemia in Pregnant African Women. The Central African Journal of Medicine 19(4): 133–136.

Lamphere, L.

1974 Strategies, Cooperation and Conflict Among Women in Domestic groups. *In* Woman, Culture and Society, M. Z. Rosaldo and L. Lamphere (eds.), Stanford: Stanford University Press.

Landy, D.

1977 Role Adaptation: Traditional Curers under the Impact of Western Medicine. *In* Culture, Disease and Healing: Studies in Medical Anthropology, D. Landy, (ed.), New York: Macmillan Publishing Co., Inc.

Last, M.

1976 The Presentation of Sickness in a Community of Non-Muslim Hausa. *In* Social Anthropology and Medicine, J. B. Loudon (ed.), San Francisco: Academic Press.

Leach, E. R.

1960 The Sinhalese of the Dry Zone of Northern Ceylon. *In* Social Structure in Southeast Asia, G. P. Murdock (ed.), Chicago: Aldine.

Lebeuf, A.

1960 Women in Political Organization. *In* Women of Tropical Africa, D. Paulme (ed.), Berkeley: University of California Press.

Leis, N. B.

1974 Women in Groups: Ijaw Women's Associations. *In* Woman, Culture and Society, M. Z. Rosaldo and L. Lamphere (eds.), Stanford, Stanford University Press.

Lingenfelter, S. G.

1977 Emic Structure and Decision-Making in Yap. Ethnology 16:351–52.

Lombard, J.

1965 Structures de Type "Féodal" en Afrique Noire. Paris and The Hague: Mouton and Co., Publishers.

Maclean, U.

1976 Some Aspects of Sickness Behaviour Among the Yoruba. *In* Social Anthropology and Medicine, J. B. Louden (ed.), London, New York, San Francisco: Academic Press.

Mati, J. K. G. and A. Hatimy

1971 The Importance of Anemia of Pregnancy in Nairobi and the Role of Malaria in the Aetiology of Megaloblastic Anaemia. Journal of Tropical Medicine and Hygiene 74(1):1–8.

McClain, C.

1975 Ethno-Obstetrics in Aijijic. Anthropological Quarterly 48(1):38–56.

Mburu, F. M.

1977 The Duality of Traditional and Western Medicine in Africa: Mystics, Myths and Reality. *In* Traditional Healing: New Science of New Colonialism, P. Singer (ed.), New York: Conch Magazine Ltd.: 158–85.

Meek, C. K.

1937 Law and Authority in a Nigerian Tribe; A Study in Indirect Rule. 1970 reprint. New York: Barnes and Noble, Inc.

Mensah-Dapaa, W. S.

1979 Observations on Traditional Healing Methods in Ghana. *In* African Therapeutic Systems. Ademuwagun et al. (eds.), Waltham: Crossroads press.

Mongeau, B. et al.

1960 The "Granny" Midwife: Changing Roles and Functions of a Folk Practitioner. The American Journal of Sociology 66:497–505.

Morsy, Soheir

In Press Childbirth in an Egyptian village. *In* An Anthology of Human Birth. M. Kay (ed.), Philadelphia: F. A. Davis.

Myles, M. F.

1975 Textbook for Midwives. Edinburgh, London and New York: Churchill Livingstone.

Naassou, M. L.
1974 Rural Midwives in Togo. Report of the Francophone West African Working Party. International Confederation of Midwives. Dakar, Senegal, November 17–23.
Neumann, A. K. et al.
1974 Traditional Birth Attendants – a Key to Rural Maternal and Child Health and Family Planning Services. Environmental Child Health, February: 21–27.
Ngubane, Harriet
1976 Some Aspects of Treatment Among the Zulu. *In* Social Anthropology and Medicine. J. Loudon (ed.), A. S. A. Monograph 13. London: Academic Press.
Olson, M., Jr.
1965 The Logic of Collective Action: Public Goods and the Theory of Groups. Cambridge: Harvard University Press.
Ortiz, S.
1967 The Structure of Decision-Making Among Indians of Colombia. *In* Themes in Economic Anthropology, R. Firth (ed.), London: Tavistock.
Osgood, K. et al.
1966 Lay Midwifery in Southern Appalachia. Archives of Environmental Health 12: 759–70.
Otoo, S. N.
1973 The Traditional Management of Puberty and Childbirth Among the Ga People, Ghana. Tropical and Geographical Medicine 15:88–94.
Paul, B. D.
1955 Health, Culture and Community: Case Studies of Public Reactions to Health Programs. New York: Russel Sage Foundation.
Paul, L.
1975 Recruitment to a Ritual Role; The Midwife in a Maya Community. Ethos 3(3): 449–67.
Paul, L. and B. D. Paul
1975 The Maya Midwife as Sacred Specialist: A Guatemalan Case. American Ethnologist 2(4):707–26.
Paulme, D.
1960 Women of Tropical Africa. Berkeley: University of California Press.
Payne, J. W.
1972 Alternative Approaches to Decision-Making Under Risk: Moments vs Risk Dimensions. Working Papers, 10. School of Social Science, University of California. Irvine.
Pillsbury, Barbara L. K.
1978 "Doing the Month": Confinement and Convalescence of Chinese Women after Childbrith. Soc. Sci. and Med. 12:11–22.
Population Reports
1980 Series J. Number 22. Traditional Midwives and Family Planning. Baltimore: The Johns Hopkins University.
Prattis, J. I.
1973 Strategising Man. Man 8(1):46–58.
Pritchard, J. A. and P. C. Macdonald
1973 Williams Obstetrics. 15th edition. New York, Appleton-Century-Grofts.
Pritchard, J. A. and P. C. Macdonald
1976 Williams Obstetrics. 15th edition. New York, Appleton-Century-Crofts.
Quinn, N.
1975 Decision Models of Social Structure. American Ethnologist 2(1):19–45.
Riley, J. N. and S. Sermsri
1974 The Variegated Thai Medical system as a Context for Birth Control Services. Working Paper No. 6. Mahidol University.

Rogers, E. M. and F. F. Shoemaker
1971 Communication of Innovations: A Cross-Cultural Approach. New York: The Free Press.

Rogers, E. M. and D. S. Solomon
1973 Traditional Midwives for Family Planning Communication in Asia. Honolulu: East-West Communication Institute.

Romanucci-Ross, L.
1969 The Hierarchy of Resort in Curative Practice: The Admiralty Islands, Melanesia. Journal of Health and Social Behavior 10:201–09.

Ronen, D.
1975 Dahomey: Between Tradition and Modernity. New York, Cornell University Press.

Rosaldo, M. Z.
1974 Woman, Culture and Society: A Theoretical Overview. *In* Woman, Culture and Society, M. Z. Rosaldo and L. Lamphere (eds.), Stanford: Stanford University Press.

Rubel, A. J. et al.
1971 Characteristics of Traditional Birth Attendants (Mananabang) in Metropolitan Cebu. *In* Culture and Population, S. Polgar (ed.), Chapel Hill, N. C.: Carolina Population Center Publication, Monograph 9.

Rubel, A. J. and Carolyn Sargout (eds.)
1979 Parallel Medical Systems: Paper From a Workshop on 'The Healing Process'. Social Science and Medicine 13B(1).

Sanday, P. R.
1974 Female Status in the Public Domain. *In* Woman, Culture and Society, M. Z. Rosaldo and L. Lamphere (ed.), Stanford: Stanford University Press.

Saunders, L.
1954 Cultural Difference and Medical Care: The Case of the Spanish-Speaking People of the Southwest. New York: Russell Sage Foundation.

Sich, Dorothea
1979 Traditional Concepts and Customs on Pregnancy, Birth and Post Partum Period in Rural Korea. Paper presented at 1st International Conference on Traditional Medicine. Camberra: Australian National University.

Simon, H. A. and A. Newell
1971 Human Problem Solving: The State of Theory in 1970. American Psychologist 26:145–59.

Slovic, P. and S. Lichtenstein
1968 Relative Importance of Probabilities and Payoffs in Risk Taking. Journal of Experimental Psychology 79(3)2.

Snow, Loudell F.
1974 Folk Medical Beliefs and Their Implications for Care of Patients. Annals of Internal Medicine 81(1):82–96.

Takpara, I.
1977 Mortalités Maternelle et Périnatale. Prévention: Solutions pour une Politique Sanitaire de Masse en Soins Obstétricaux en République Populaire du Bénin. These de doctorat en Médicine.

Thibaut, J. W. and H. H. Kelly
1959 The Social Psychology of Groups. New York: Wiley.

Thompson, B. and D. Baird
1967a Some Impressions of Childbearing in Tropical Areas. Part I. Journal of Obstetrics and Gynecology of the British Commonwealth 74:329–38.

Thompson, B. and D. Baird
1967b Some Impressions of Childbearing in the Tropical Areas. Part II. Pre-eclampsia

and Low Birthweight. Journal of Obstetrics and Gynecology of the British Commonwealth 74:499–509.

Thompson, B. and D. Baird
1967c Some Impressions of Childbearing in Tropical Areas. Part III. Outcome of Labor. Journal of Obstetrics and Gynecology of the British Commonwealth, 74:510–522.

Turner, V. W.
1968 The Drums of Affliction. Oxford: Clarendon Press.

Van Allen, J.
1976 African Women, "Modernization" and National Liberation. *In* Women in the World: A Comparative Study, L. B. Iglitzgin and R. Ross (eds.), Santa Barbara: Clio Books.

Van Baal, J.
1971 Symbols for Communication. Assen: Van Gorcum and Co.

Verderese, Maria de Lourdes and Lily M. Turnbull
1975 The Traditional Birth Attendant in Maternal and Child Health and Family Planning. Geneva: World Health Organization.

Warren, D. M.
1978 The Interpretation of Change in a Ghanaian Ethnomedical Study. Human Organization 37(1):74–77.

Wolff, B. B. and S. Langley
1968 Cultural Factors and the Response to Pain: A Review. American Anthropologist 70:494–501.

Wolff, N. H.
1979 Concepts of Causation and Treatment in the Yoruba Medical System: The Special Case of Barrenness. *In* African Therapeutic Systems, Ademuwagun et al. (eds.), Waltham: Crossroads Press.

World Health Organization
1979 Traditional Birth Attendants. World Health Organization Publication No. 44. Geneva.

Young, A.
1976 Some Implications of Medical Beliefs and Practices for Social Anthropology. American Anthropologist 78:5–24.

Zaltman, G. and R. Duncan
1977 Strategies for Planned Change. New York: Wiley.

Zborowski, M.
1969 People in Pain. San Francisco: Jossey-Bass.

INDEX

abiku 29, 113
abnormal births 90, 91, 116, 118, 120
abortifacients 41
abortion 40, 41
  Bariba concepts regarding 35, 42
access to information, correlation with social class 12
accomodation, in medical systems 163, 164
Adama Worou 112–114, 125, 132
adultery, and obstetrical complications 26, 34, 116
African midwifery 157
age, as status attribute of midwives 62, 64, 70
age structure, in Pehunko 168
agriculture 137, 138
Alihonou, E. 8, 106, 135, 149–151, 155
amniotic sac 107, 114, 122
ampoule 27
anemia 149–151
apprenticeship 104, 109
  of midwives 62, 65, 67–69
aristocrats 44, 45, 47, 50, 61, 66, 104, 114
associations, of women 48, 49
Atakora province 155
attributes, of matrones 83, 114, 120, 158
avoidance 71, 97

baby-washers 72, 76, 77
baby-washing 96, 100, 101, 112, 122
Bariba 3–5, 50
  as civil servants 12
  cosmology 19
  restriction of activities 8
  society 43
baptism 45
behavior, and prediction 146
Benin clinics *see also* district clinic
Benin clinics 151, 152
birth
  as an event 87
  definition of 86, 88, 89, 92, 95, 140
birth assistance 88
  choice of 145, 146, 156
  patterns of 96, 97, 142
birth attendant 63, 81, 103
birth setting 111
bleeding 106, 108, 122, 123, 133, 151, 155
Bona 120–123, 132, 133
bori 77
boundary maintenance behavior 143, 144
breach of taboo 27, 116
breast abcess 155
breathing exercises 130
breech birth 106, 120, 131, 143
budgeting priorities 154, 155
bukakaaru 77–79, 81
bureaucracy 142
burial 30, 109

Caesarian section 150, 156
census 5, 168
  of matrones 63
character attributes, of midwives 79, 81, 82
child care 74, 75
childbirth training 128–130
childhood illnesses 70, 75
chronology of the delivery process 106
circumcision 36, 46, 71
  female 35, 37, 46, 54, 75, 103, 150, 169, 170
civil service 13
civil servants 17, 134–138, 140, 142, 143, 159, 166
clairvoyance 77, 81
class distinctions 165
client-practioner interactions 62, 111, 158
clinic delivery 91, 134–139, 141, 142, 149, 158
  morbidity 147, 153
  mortality 147, 149, 153
clinic patients, attributes of 134, 135, 137, 138, 143, 158
clinic records 134, 135, 137, 138
clinic use 137–144*ff.*, 156, 161, 162
  morbidity 151
  mortality 151
clinical reality 93–95
  and birth assistance 132
  models of 16, 95, 132, 160–163, 166
clitoridectomy 35, 37, 46, 54, 75, 103, 150, 169, 170
collaboration, between matrones 104, 114, 117–119, 166
commerce 72, 136
commoners 44, 45, 66, 104
communication, and clinic use 138, 139

competence
  and age 98
  in obstetrics 158
complications of labor 76, 150, 156, 161
comprehensive care, by matrones 74, 75
conception 54
  Bariba ideas regarding 35, 37, 38, 41, 42
contagion 28
contraception 39, 40
  Bariba ideas regarding 38
cord-cutting 96, 97, 99–101, 112, 122, 124
cord traction 153
Cosminsky, S. 63, 72
cosmology 19
cosmopolitan medical personnel 151, 154, 155, 159, 161, 166
cosmopolitan medical services 1, 124, 154
cosmopolitan medicine 94, 96, 97, 99, 111, 115–119, 123, 124, 127, 133, 143, 156, 159, 164–166
costs 13, 15, 142, 144
  and decision-making 144–146
courage 99, 112–114, 120, 127, 128, 142, 145, 158, 162
credit associations 48
cross-cultural study of midwifery 93, 105, 157–159
cultivators 135, 136, 138
cults 77–82
cupping 33
cursing, and sterility 41, 42
cystoceles 117

decisions, and obstetrical assistance 86, 95
decision-making
  and authority among co-wives 51
  and costs 144–146
  and responsibility 52, 132
  and role expectations 62, 82
  and witchcraft beliefs 95
  factors influencing 146, 157, 163
  in agriculture 47
  patterns of 136, 137
  womens' roles in 52–54, 157
decision-making process 35, 132
delivery 54, 56, 87–89, 124, 161
  as performance 124
  complications 161
  ideal behavior during 96, 128–131, 162
  obstructed 106, 107, 117, 150, 156
  role of men 133
  stillbirth 115
delivery assistance 113
  category of 97, 98
  patterns of 96–102, 105, 117, 120, 123, 131–133, 142
  preferences for 143, 144, 156–158, 161
  reasons for 96
  selection of 118
delivery goals 13, 96, 144, 146, 158
delivery outcome 133, 147, 156
delivery position 91, 94, 121, 150, 151, 166
delivery strategies 13
diagnosis 24, 86
  and divination 59
  Bariba concepts regarding 160
  decisions regarding 34
  of pregnancy 75
diet, post-partum 123
diffusion of innovations 10
disease causation 28, 59
dispensary 115, 118, 121, 133–137, 146
dissociation, and pain 130
distance
  and clinic use 138–140
  and delivery 141
district clinic 6, 134–144, 150, 156
  utilization of 7
divination 28, 30, 77, 78, 80, 106
divining
  and sickness 29
  and status of women 54
  and treatment of sterility 75
diviners 28, 29, 59
  as sterility specialists 41
divorce 50, 53
Djerma 98
Dogi 113
Doh 102–105
  birth assistants 103
  neighborhoods 103
domestic domain 43, 46
domestic relations 50
domestic unit 47
dreams, in healing 70
drugs 155, 165
Dutch medicine 130
dysmenorrhea 122

eclampsia 153
economic subsistence 47
edema 117, 119, 162
education 144
  as status attribute of midwives 62, 64
efficacy 1, 15, 16, 86, 92, 146, 156, 160, 163

elite 165
emic perspective 155
episiotomy 150
estimated date of delivery 106
ethnicity 165
etic perspective 147
evacuation, of patients 153

family allocation 142
family origin, as status attribute of midwives 66
family status, as status attribute of midwives 62, 65
fatigue, of parturients 108, 155
features of clients 17
features of the decision-making process 17
features of the disorder 17
female responsibility 158
female specialists 157, 158
fertility 45
 and Bariba values 42
fetal presentation 90, 92, 93, 106, 107, 143
fetus 161
 Bariba concepts regarding 38, 39
fever 155
folk syndrome 119
food taboos 87, 123, 131
Foster, G. 2, 9
Fulbe 66, 98, 138
fumigation 162
 medicines used in 33

gossip 135, 136, 140
government health services
 quality of care 154
 use of 134, 137, 138, 156
government midwives 64, 83, 84, 91, 93, 116, 141, 158, 161, 165
government policy 144, 157, 158
gusunɔ̃ 19
gynecological products 155

Hausa 98, 114, 116
healers 45, 56, 57, 59, 61, 103
 apprenticeship 56, 58, 65
 categories of 58–61
 characteristics of 62
collaboration between 104, 114, 117–119, 165
 power of 56, 59, 60
healing 124
 and diagnosis 24
 and possession 80, 81
 and symptom presentation 24
 efficacy of 92
 techniques of 30
 women as 61
health care decision-making *see also* decision-making
health care decision-making 1
 and construction of clinical reality 16
 and efficacy 15
 Bariba data 11
 concept of relative advantage 10
 cultural logic of 19
 features of the process 17
 multi-factor model 10
 obstetrical care choices 9, 15
 relative costs 10
 responsibility for 14
 single-factor models 9
health care planning 160
health infrastructure 144
hemoglobin 149, 150
hemorrhage 133, 151, 153
hemorrhoids 107, 117
Heath, A. 10
herbalist 59
hereditary occupations 61, 76
heterophily 15, 62
hierarchy of assistance 105, 109
home delivery 134, 149, 150, 151, 156, 158, 166
 morbidity 147, 150, 151, 153
 mortality 147, 151, 153
homophily 15, 16, 62–64, 84, 158, 160, 163
household
 women's responsibilities in 51, 52
 composition of 98, 168
human nature, Bariba conception of 21
hunters 128
hypnosis 129

ideal behavior during labor 96, 128–131, 133, 141, 162
ideological orientation, of national government 144
illness of pregnancy *see also* pregnancy, complications of
illnesses of pregnancy 87
impotence 2, 30, 41, 42
incantations 59, 60
indigenous healers, in national health planning 1, 159, 160, 165

indigeneous midwives *see also* matrones
indigenous midwives 93
  collaboration between 166
  integration into national health plans 159–160, 164, 165
  training of 163–165
infant mortality 113
infanticide 90, 91, 120, 143
infection 151, 154
information, and clinic use 138, 139, 143, 159
ingestion, of medicines 33
inheritance, by women 49
injection 116, 123, 127
interviewing *see also* methodology
interviewing 105, 106
  of matrones 63
intrauterine death 106, 107, 115
iron supplementation 150
Islam 3, 45

Janzen, J. 13, 14, 132
Jordan, B. 8, 9, 93, 94, 130

Kentucky midwives 105
kinship
  and baby-washing 101
  and birth assistance 100
  and cord-cutting 101
Kleinman, A. 16, 93, 132
koru water 122, 127
Kouande 2, 134, 137, 138, 140, 143, 156, 157, 163, 165, 166
  population statistics 138

labor 54, 88, 89, 105, 106, 113, 121, 140, 162
  and pain 124–131*ff.*
  complications of 161
  delayed 106–109, 121
  ideal behavior during 96, 128–131, 133, 141, 162
  induction of 107
  obstructed 106, 107, 114, 150, 156
  pushing 115
lacerations 106, 108
Lamaze 128
language, and delivery assistance 114
lithotomy position 94
Lombard, J. 3, 53, 74

Maclean, U. 2
magic 30
  sympathetic 112, 115, 121, 124
male responsibility 50
manual techniques, in delivery 108
marital relations 52, 53
marital status, as status attribute of midwives 62, 65
marketing, government influence on 144
marriage 50, 51, 66
maternal and child health care 1
maternal morbidity 149
  causes of 150
maternal mortality 90, 147, 149, 152
  in Benin 152, 154
matrones 63–65, 68, 81
  as healers 81
  attributes of 83, 104, 114, 120, 158
  integration of, into national health services 159, 160, 164
  of Doh 103
  prototype 82, 83
  role of 88
  recruitement 68
  status characteristics of 74, 104
Mata 130
Mayan midwives 105
Mburu, E. 56, 59
medical models 160–163
medical practitioners, and "medicine people" 56
medical resources, and health planning policy 165
medicines 32, 33, 57–60, 65, 68
  Bariba 116, 117
  for delivery 112, 115–117, 121, 132
  for pain 126
  homeopathic 32
medicine person 58, 59, 61, 73, 76, 80, 81
membranes 107, 112, 114
menopause 61, 64, 65, 71
  Bariba concepts regarding 35, 38
menstruation 2, 36, 37, 50, 65, 131
  Bariba concepts regarding 35, 37
methodology 63, 96, 105, 106
  interviewing, in Kouande 6, 7
  interviewing, of possession cult members 8
  medical collaboration 8
  use of census 5
midwife
  and status of women 54
  apprenticeship 65–69
  as a category 61
  as a family specialty 67
  as a female activity 46
  as a female professional specialty 56

midwife (*continued*)
as healer 60, 62, 63
as hereditary occupation 61
as medicine person 61
as part-time specialty 72
definition of 63
position of 56
midwifery
as a therapeutic system 2, 96, 105, 109, 110
as a skill 61
as source of income 72
cross-cultural studies 8, 83, 84
shared concepts of 110
transmission of skills 76
techniques and practices 9, 39, 105, 106, 109-111, 118, 120, 122, 126
midwives
attributes 8, 15, 62-64, 79, 82, 84, 114, 158
categorization of 56, 63, 64
functions of 56
in Kentucky 105
integration into national health system 8, 159, 160, 164
inteviewing 5, 63, 105, 106
Mayan 105
power of 60
status of 8, 54, 73, 84, 104
misfortune 158
major causes of 89
model of health service utilization 144
assumptions underlying 16
features of 17
modesty 71, 116, 119, 141-143, 145, 162
morality, Bariba concepts regarding 19
morbidity 134, 165
and emic view 155, 156
Morsy, S. 94
mortality 134, 148, 165
among children 151, 169
and emic view 155, 156
maternal 147
perinatal 151
multipara 107, 136

national government 144, 147, 158
national health care planning 155, 159, 160
and national integration 144, 159, 160
and national priorities 154, 155, 165
national health care system 159, 160, 165
role of indifenous healers 1, 159-161*ff.*
neighborhoods *see also* Pehunko
neighborhoods 99-102, 114
Nicole 131, 133
nutritional deficiencies 149

obstetrical auxiliaries 163, 164
obstetrical care, defined 1
obstetrical care choices 159, 160
obstetrical care decision-making *see also* decision-making, health care decision-making
obstetrical care decision-making 15, 35
hypotheses regarding 16, 17
preferences, and efficacy 86-95*ff.*
obstetrical complications 24, 26, 34, 38, 86, 92, 106, 124, 131, 132, 137, 138, 150, 151, 154, 156-158, 161
obstetrical emergencies 132, 137, 138, 143, 153, 156
obstetrical medicines *see also* medicines
obstetrical medicines 33, 38
obstetrical techniques and practices *see also* midwifery techniques and practices
obstetrical techniques and practices 164
obstetrics, cross-cultural study of 83, 84, 157
obstructed delivery *see also* complications of labor
obstructed delivery 150, 151, 156
occupation, as status attribute of midwifes 66

pain 111-114, 123, 127
and childbirth education 128, 129
and courage 127, 129
and fear 126
and reality 126
and shame 126, 129
and socialization 127, 129
cross-cultural studies 129, 130
cultural dimension 125, 126, 130
experience of 125, 128, 129
expression of 124, 128, 130
in childbirth 126-131 passim, 162
measurement of 125, 129, 130
medication for 126
physiological dimension 126
responses to 125-128
parallel health care systems 1
Parkia biglobosa 108, 121
patient-practitioner encounters 132

patient-practitioner relationship 93, 94, 96
Paul, L. 65
peasants 159, 165
Pehunko 3, 63
demographic data 6
economy 5
neighborhoods 96–102, 135, 168
pelvic disproportion 151
perinatal mortality 151
Pillsbury, B. 94
pharmacies 155
pharmacopeia *see also* medicines
pharmacopeia 24, 39, 56, 166
placenta 39, 89, 97, 105, 108, 109, 112, 114, 117, 118, 122, 124, 139, 151, 153, 156, 160, 161
poisoner 58
political positions 49
polygamy 51–53
population statistics 138, 168
possession
among men 78
and divination 80
cults 77–82, 119
initiation into cults 78–82
possession spirits 20
inheritance of 79
post-partum complications 106, 108, 151
post-partum diet 123
power 23, 24, 80
praise-singing 61, 73, 79
pregnancy 56, 75, 87, 106, 131, 149
and status of women 54
Bariba concepts regarding 24, 26, 27, 34
diagnosis 75
high risk 88
ideal behavior during 87, 88
knowledge of 87
prematurity 111, 113
prenatal consultations 123, 135, 136, 149, 150, 155
primipara 96, 107, 129, 130, 135, 136
prolapsed cord 116–120, 124, 133, 162
prolapsed uterus 117
proverbs 53
psychological support 116, 166
public domain 46
defined 43
puerperal fever 150
pushing, during labor 115, 121

'rabit' 28
rational choice theory 10, 12, 15
rationality 146, 147, 156, 161
recruitment, of midwives 62, 67, 68
rectoceles 117
referral system 165, 166
regionalism 165
religion 19
as status attribute of midwives 62, 63
renumeration 71, 72
of midwives 62
reproduction 43, 157
as domain of women 54, 55
disorders 56
ideal constructs of 35
reproductive complex 158
reproductive goals 157
reproductive history 111, 113
of matrones 70
residence
and baby-washing 101, 102
and birth assistance 100
and birth attendants 102
and clinic use 138, 139
and cord-cutting 102
and delivery preferences 140, 141
and prenatal consultations 140
as status attribute of midwives 62–64
retained placenta 76
role expectations 62–66*ff*., 86, 158
and decision-making 62, 82
for birth assistance 62
role models 143, 159
role variability, of matrones 62, 76
Rosaldo, M. 43

Sako 114–116, 132, 133
salt 119
sambani 77–81
sample size *see* methodology
Sanday, P. 43
scarring, as treatment 33
sex education 36, 51
sex roles 44–55 passim, 158
sexual relations, and power of medicines 65
shame 53, 97, 114, 115, 129
shaming 116
shea butter 47
Sich, D. 94
sickness causation 23, 34, 158, 160
and breach of taboo 27, 34
attribution of responsibility 21
Bariba concept regarding 19, 25, 33, 62

slaves 66, 113
soaking, medicines for 33
social control 116
socialization 127, 129
solitary delivery 85, 91, 96–99, 105, 124, 143, 157, 158
sorcery 21, 22, 29–31, 33, 70
  and complications of pregnancy 26, 27, 34
  as cause of sterility 41
source of healing knowledge 69
spirits 20, 23
  and apprenticeship 58
  and midwives 62
  of the bush 77
spirit possession 50, 77–82
  frequency 78
  symptoms 80
spirit possession cults 8, 46, 53, 104
  and diviners 28
  and status of women 54
  interviews with members 8
'squirrel' 28
status, and titles 45, 49, 61
status, of women 45, 158
  and professional specialization 54
status characteristics of midwives 63–67
status differentiation 160
sterility 2, 88
  Bariba concepts regarding 35, 41, 42
  treatment 75, 76
sterility specialists 42, 54, 103
stillbirth 115
stoicism 113, 125, 128, 130
stratification 44, 46, 160
substances *see also* medicines
substances 59, 60
support services 144
symbolic gestures, mused by matrones 124
symptom interpretation 24, 114, 116, 119, 160–163

Takpara, I. 151, 153
tamabu 58
tetanus 155
therapeutic options *see also* decision-making, health care decision-making
therapeutic options 8, 19, 110, 156, 157, 160
  single-factor models 9
tigpiru 25, 26, 107–109, 116, 117, 119, 122, 131, 155, 156, 162
titles 45, 49, 61
  inheritance 45
traders 48, 49, 72, 134, 135, 138, 144, 159
training programs 63, 164, 165
transportation 137, 142, 144, 145
transverse presentation 106, 118
tribute 73, 74
twins 118, 132

urbanism 142
urban elite 144
utilization of national health services 134–156*ff*.

vaginal examinations 107, 108
values, and clinic utilization 142–145
vertigo 155
village size, and number of matrones 104

warriors 128
washing, medicine for 33
weddings 45
witch babies 89–92, 109, 111, 113, 120, 142, 143, 162
  and delivery 91, 92
witchcraft 23, 70, 82, 93, 95, 109, 113, 131, 157
  and pregnancy complications 26, 34
women
  and power 50
  authority of 46
  as healers 45
  as traders 48, 49
  role of 1, 46, 47, 115
  status of 43, 44, 53, 54
women of reproductive age 100, 155–157
  and selection of birth assistance, survey of 46, 96–98, 134, 168
  ages of women in study 6
  census 6
  interviewing of 5
words 81
  and medicines 58–60
World Health Organization 152

Yaayi Bore 116–122 passim
Yaayi Ganigi 111–115 passim
Yaayi Yo 117–119 passim
Yon Sika 120, 132
Young, A. 92

Zborowski, M. 125, 127